MARTIN C. SCHULTZ

Indiana University

An Analysis of Clinical Behavior in Speech and Hearing

Prentice-Hall, Inc., Englewood Cliffs, N.J.

© 1972 by Prentice-Hall, Inc., Englewood Cliffs, N. J.

Library of Congress Catalog Card Number: 70-37024

Printed in the United States of America

ISBN:
0-13-032920-7

10   9   8   7   6   5   4   3   2   1

Prentice-Hall International, Inc., *London*
Prentice-Hall of Australia, Pty. Ltd., *Sydney*
Prentice-Hall of Canada, Ltd., *Toronto*
Prentice-Hall of India Private Limited, *New Delhi*
Prentice-Hall of Japan, Inc., *Tokyo*

Contents

Preface

This book presents a model of the clinical decision process in speech and hearing. The reader is asked to judge the presentation by its success in dealing with two questions of concern to him: Does the book offer insight into the methodology of clinical activities? and, Does the model provide a workable base for becoming clinically competent? In other words, we have proposed to deal with the methodology of the field. This is to be a reference book for the student or practitioner, intended to increase his understanding of, and thereby his confidence in, the procedures he uses, to help him choose clinical tactics to adopt with particular patients, and the like.

Does the field need a presentation of clinical methodology and, if so, why by a speech and hearing scientist? I think the answer to the first part of the question is that there is a significant need. I am trying to give the beginning student in clinical practice an organizing scheme to assist his learning because I think he is, on the average, overwhelmed by the task he faces. We ask the student arriving at the stage of initial clinical contact to learn a wide variety of things, to learn them well, and to do it in a hurry. We are asking him to become sensitive to observations and perceptions that are important in understanding his patients, though he may not yet fully understand what he should look for. We are asking that he become sensitive to procedures to modify the communication behaviors of others in some lasting way, when he may be only grossly aware of what motivates any behavior in any human being, himself included. At a time when we are typically burdening our student with a myriad of particular skills to be experienced and mastered, we would like him also to have sufficient detachment to see the "grander scheme" of why we do X, how it relates to Y, and why it should precede Z.

I further believe that probably only someone unencumbered with clinical duties, and perhaps free of clinical teaching, can do the job. I assert there is reason that so many researchers are continually fuming and fussing about clinical problems, with which they may personally never deal, whereas so few clinicians seem to raise the same kind of fuss. The reason lies in the nature of the breeds. Researchers seem conditioned to thinking "group" thoughts and concern themselves with groups clinicians consider large even when the experimenter occupies himself with what he considers small samples. Clinicians, a different species, look at people one at a time. They are less taken with the problems of the group and more intimately involved in the intricacy of detail that makes each patient unique. Experimentalists, perhaps, tend to be more macroscopic and clinicians microscopic in approach.

At least in the present instance the general statement seems to apply. This book is a macroscopic view of clinical decision processes, in the sense that few specific suggestions will be found. Even without being a working clinician, I subscribe to the rule that nobody desires to prescribe therapy in absentia. Over and above this, I am not trying to alter the microscopic anatomy of evaluation, therapy, teaching, or research. Rather, this book is the anatomy of the "grander scheme."

Many persons have contributed to my ideas as expressed in these pages. I owe each and all, teachers, colleagues, and students, a debt I cannot begin to describe or repay. Dana Main, formerly with the Sensory Intelligence Laboratory, The University of Michigan, was largely responsible for my original formulation of the model presented. Marilyn Berman, now a fellow faculty member at Indiana University, was also a member of that Lab's staff during the early discussions of the model and made significant original contributions to my thinking (for which she might receive some credit but should not be chastised). As many readers will be aware, the model grows out of statistical decision theory and some of the sophistication of these ideas developed in the Theory of Signal Detectability. During the summer of 1966 Wilson P. (Spike) Tanner, Jr., Director of the Sensory Intelligence Laboratory, served as a mentor and guide during my early struggles to wrestle a structure out of decision theory that might be applicable to "things clinical," and he has been a constant source of guidance and deeply insightful intelligence.

Several friends and colleagues were kind enough to put up with reading the manuscript and giving more extensive comments on earlier versions. Charles D. Parker and Allan J. Heffler were instrumental in causing me to continue beyond my original efforts. Sophie Hadjian and Betty Mintz tried, too often unsuccessfully, to make me appreciate the depths of my clinical naivete. Edgar R. Garrett and Jean and Kay Rigg made me realize in a most dramatic way the impact that some of the newer technologies would have on the clinical profession. Mary Carpenter worked through the manuscript alone and with some thoughtful students to try to help me appreciate the difference between what I had written and what should be done to make the book more meaningful to students, and to her and Rona Alexander, Connie Lautner, and Mary Jo Steckol I offer much thanks.

Bob Dunn made me aware repeatedly, with style and gusto, of the debt I owe him as editor and friend.

Finally, it is a pleasure gratefully to acknowledge the support of the Indiana University Foundation. The Foundation twice awarded me Summer Faculty Fellowships to allow time for my studies and writing. To my wife Beatrice no statement, public or private, can begin to give appropriate credit.

MARTIN C. SCHULTZ

Bloomington, Indiana

ONE

Introduction

We begin the book by dealing with the needs of a student entering his first course in clinical practice. Anyone in a new learning experience, which includes complex multiple aspects, needs to learn to establish priorities, enabling him to reduce his errors and function successfully.

The beginning student must learn what to observe and then observe carefully; he must learn to separate description from inference; he must learn to conduct himself in a professional and ethical manner; he must learn how to define goals and procedures, separate them, and employ them discriminatingly and with poise. In essence, what the student needs is the personal guidance and advice of a masterful supervising clinician. Unfortunately, few if any training programs can provide a continuous flow of clinical wisdom for each student. We address ourselves in this book to meeting some of the needs of the student in each of these experiences.

Our approach is based on the assumption that there is a recognizable methodology common to supervising clinicians responsible for transmitting clinical wisdom to each new generation of professionals. We will deal with such questions as when therapy should be applied and when it might be wasted effort, and what types of information are required in an evaluation. Excellent discussions of evaluative procedures, therapy materials, recording forms, and appropriate equipment are available, so we will concern ourselves with none of these matters.[1] Our concern can be thought of as structuring the clinical decisions that are the responsibility of any clinician, so we begin with a discussion of the clinician as information processor or as decision maker.

---

[1] A large number of specific subject areas will be covered in the sections following. A bibliography that includes most topics appears at the end of the manuscript, organized by subject matter.

The Clinician as Decision Maker

The clinician going about his daily activities can be viewed as an information processing system. Although the operation is not understood, the basic elements in processing information can be described. Information processing systems use two sources of information for their task: the first is external, which we will call *observation;* [2] the other is internal, comprising *memory.* Memory-derived knowledge has been at some time observed, after which it undergoes complex processing—abstracting, classifying, and labeling—and it will be helpful to keep in mind the distinction between immediately experienced and memory-derived inputs to the processor. What one does in processing information is to combine observations and memories to draw conclusions or inferences about the things observed. In a formal manner, this involves a procedure for operating upon (or making decisions about) the information according to some internal set of rules. The processor somehow combines the observations and memories to reach decisions about the things observed, but the exact procedures elude us.

If I am asked to think of a chair, I can do so in great detail. I can see a specific chair, remember what it feels like to touch it, how heavy it is to lift, and many other particulars. I can do this for many chairs that I remember. What I cannot do is think about a general category of chairs without dealing with specific properties of specific chairs. I can only recall from memory *particular* chairs, not the general class. On the other hand, I have no difficulty in retrieving individual chairs from my memory without getting tables or snowflakes mixed in, so I must somehow have stored a general category of chairs in my memory bank as a label pinned to many specific memories.

The relationships among specific memories and general classes in memory are not understood. I would speculate that the ability to deal with a general class in some ways but not in others results from the kind of label we affix to perceptions. These labels are the addresses we assign to the perceptions, and these addresses are subsequently used to recall the memory. The implication of label-as-address is that if I do not label some part of an observation I may not be able to recall it—if I do not consider something important enough to assign a name to it, I may never put it into permanent memory.

[2] We will use the term "observation" for any sense-experienced input. It need not be visual or even restricted to a single sensory mechanism.

To restate this point in terms of the example of the chairs, if I routinely sit on a coffee table in my living room, I may also think of it as a "chair" and may recall it when thinking of chairs, but I will recall it as a chair precisely because I perceive (label) it as a chair. Yet I may get in and out of my car several times a day for months but not be able to recall if there is a brand name on the car radio because I have never thought it important to store that information.

The parts of the decision process (information processing procedure) that we do not understand reside in answers to such questions as: How does one address his own memory? Why do we recall from memory the particular perceptions that we combine with the immediate observation and why do we not recall other aspects? How does the combination of memory portions and observation patterns occur? What are we doing when we draw inferences? What are the specifics of the task? Summarily, what are the rules by which the system operates? All of these are elusive questions and probably will remain so.

On the other hand, some parts of the decision process are relatively simple to understand, in spite of our difficulty in comprehending the operation of the portions of the central nervous system they involve. We shall use the same description or model repeatedly to deal with them, for it is precisely this description that forms the focus of the book.

The description of the decision process must explain what external observations are to be used and what sorts of knowledge one needs to draw from memory (even though we don't know how such material is brought from storage to a processing location). Then it must explain what one seems to do in combining the observations with the memories of the general class (which seem to be a collection of a large number of specifics that have been labeled as having common elements and are recalled individually but thought of collectively) to draw some conclusions about the thing being observed so that the conclusions have predictive value.

The text is organized to introduce the reader to some characteristics of models and modeling as a framework for evaluating the model used throughout the book. Next the model itself is developed through presentation of three clinical examples quite disparate in nature but all susceptible to description by use of the same model. Subsequent chapters deal respectively with the implications of the model for training, for clinical service in speech and in hearing, and for research in clinical processes and clinical phenomena.

The model presented below is one of an information processor–decision maker. I will delineate the components necessary to various types of clinical decisions, meanwhile repeatedly indicating how the model remains a constant factor while the specific knowledge required for a particular decision differs. *In dealing with the model we deal with a set of rules* illustrating the relationships existing among components of clinical decisions. My goal in the presentations that follow is to convince the reader that the model is useful, insightful, and open to multiple application—therefore worth learning. But the model offers no explanation of what happens in a clinical situation, or what should happen clinically. The model is the common structure but not the content of clinical activities. It is merely a model.

Models

There are several kinds of models. One type is a representation of something, altered in size, such as a scale model of a house or a greatly enlarged model of a complex molecule. Other models represent ideal forms, as a model political order, model law, or model constitution, none of which is necessarily attainable in the world of practical politics.[3] A moment's reflection will make most of us aware that mathematics tends to be the base of most of the models we use in the everyday world because it allows us to deal with complex relationships in a condensed manner.

Consider some common examples. We need not built an actual house to see if the walls will support the roof; we build a mathematical model. We quickly, and without physical effort, experiment to learn "what would happen (to the roof) if . . .". We calculate from still another model based on weather reports, geography, soil conditions, etc., what the expected snow loads or wind velocities will be; we estimate the weight and thrust the roof must bear and whatever else concerns the architect. Each consideration of roof design brings some advantages and some disadvantages, and one must evaluate each in consideration with the others to reach his decisions on design and lumber needs. But all of it is decided by using models, not buildings.

One more example may help our understanding of the nature of models. What takes place when one considers whether to go from Chicago to San Francisco by the northern or the southern route? We can easily trace the alternatives in a road atlas (another model), de-

[3] For an insightful presentation of models and modeling, see May Brodbeck, "Models, Meaning and Theories," in *Symposium on Sociological Theory*, Llewellyn Gross, (ed.) (Evanston: Row, Peterson, 1959).

termine the advantages and disadvantages of each alternative, and reach a decision. If we find, after driving too long one day, that there is a hundred-mile detour before the next gas station, we might be upset with the model maker even though we know a model does not necessarily contain everything in the original. If it were to have everything, we would no longer have a model, but an exact duplicate.

A model should include all considerations important to the decisions one expects to have based upon it and should exclude all the minor factors that could obscure the issue. Of course it may be an arbitrary decision as to what is of major and minor importance in the process or state of nature being modeled, so a model may be neither ideal nor even adequate in what it includes and excludes. A model may also be adequate for some purposes and not for others.

At this point it would be helpful to consider one fundamental attribute of all mathematical, scientific, or inductive models of any type. The relationship between such models and the state of the world they represent may be very complex, and all models are only *approximations* of the world-state. And too, determinations made by human beings are always subject to human error.[4] A designer must always provide a safety factor to compensate for differences between obtained values and average (modeled) values. The designer of a bridge or an electric motor knows that his mathematical laws are models and that in reality his model will only approximate his structure. Because the mathematical model is so precise and the real world seems so approximate, it may seem more appropriate to say that the world approximates the model, but such an orientation reflects our conditioning to a model as an ideal. One must keep in mind that reality takes precedence, so the model approximates the world.

Criteria for a Model

If it is possible to have a model that does not include all important details or that obscures them with too many superfluous details, and if it is possible to have a model that assigns too much importance to some considerations and too little to others, can we discover the criteria of a good model?

The sole yardstick of merit for a model is that of *utility*. If a model

---

[4] The complexity of relationships that may exist between models and the processes they represent is given formal recognition in Leo Apostel's "Towards the Formal Study of Models in the Non-Formal Sciences," in *The Concept and the Role of the Model in Mathematics and Natural and Social Sciences* (Dordrecht, Holland: Reidel Publishing Co., 1961), pp. 1–37.

is useful, it is good. On the other hand, if it allows some "what would happen if . . ." conclusions but not others, then it must be used with caution while a better model is sought. Inevitably most models prove to be less than adequate for some purpose, and must be discarded for better models. All our theories, in this sense, are models, and at some point must be discarded for better ones. In the interim models serve us with a power directly related to their utility and explanatory insight for for us. Expanding our control of clinical processes by use of a model shall be our purpose in the material that follows.

A second criterion for a good model might be simplicity. In constructing any model we must strip unnecessary detail and reveal the basic (and simple?) structure. However while it is true that the more simple the structure the wider its potential applicability, there is, unfortunately, the risk that it may be too unsophisticated to be a reasonable analogue for things as complex as clinical problems. So let us for a moment reserve judgment about a simplicity criterion and make the decision as we proceed in our study.

Our Model

The form of model I will use is an analogue—a simplified analogy having the important features of whatever is modeled, but with superficial and obscuring detail stripped away. Our model is essentially content-free in that we will use it to show how decisions about clinical processes can be made without detailing specific decisions. We can do this because our model is a set of rules. Specific examples of clinical decisions will be given in the development of the model in the hope that they will prove insightful for the reader, but the focus will always be on the model organizing each example, because the same model is used repeatedly and has wide potential for use in other situations. The reader should realize that this model does not have a limitless range. It is designed to spotlight certain kinds of clinical decisions to show how they are subject to a single set of rules.

While I prefer to make no judgment about a general criterion of simplicity in modeling, I assert that the great power of our clinical decision model is related to its simplicity. The simple model can be applied in situation after situation to give the clinician predictors or expectations he would not have without a model.

The same "model" a bridge engineer uses for his bridge can be used in determining what size walls are required to hold up a roof—our first example. The raw materials now become a space to be spanned, some building materials, consideration of snow or rain load (a model based on previous weather history because we think of history as a model), and the same mathematical system. If we think about the roof-building task the same way we think about the bridge-building task, our thinking pattern structures the way we perceive our raw materials. Had we used a different model, we might have labeled our raw materials differently and perceived the problem itself as being different.

Because clinicians make predictions with reasonable accuracy, I assert that they have models. Our present concern is whether or not the same model could be used in a wide variety of clinical decision processes and whether or not a single model of general applicability could be used by most clinicians. If we can demonstrate such applicability for a single model, it becomes irrelevant whether it is exactly the model clinicians use, because it is one they *can* use.

This entire text asserts that new clinicians can use a single model as a way of organizing the rules they will later follow in various clinical activities. A single model should help them realize what kind of clinical observations they must learn to make and allow them to evaluate their own progress in attaining clinical efficiency. There may be much argument against this statement concerning decisions of a clinical nature, for behind much current training seems to be a belief that "good clinicians are born," and that training can sharpen potential clinical skills but it cannot develop them. Part of this belief is that clinical skill has some underlying mystique which, while recognizable, is too elusive or complex or mysterious to be taught. This book is founded on the premise that one can present the structure of clinical decisions simply and economically so that the student can see the structure and learn it.

Organization of the Book

The work is presented in four sections. The first section develops the basic analogy, pointing up the components open to manipulation and evaluation, and some features of the various clinical processes they can be said to model. The subsequent sections deal with the applications of the model in the three divisions of the total speech and hearing profession: clinical service activities, professional training, and research.

As will be discussed in later sections, the model has sufficient generality to delineate directions for clinical research from several points of view, particularly in establishing normative data necessary but not available. Further, the model is appropriate for evaluating the growing competence of therapists-in-training, and also appropriate for determining whether they are ready to function in an independent professional capacity.

Hopefully, none of the sections of the book can be considered comprehensive, because if the analogy is to prove useful, each clinician should find applications giving him insights not even suggested by the author. We will try to show both microscopic and macroscopic views of our problem-complex. The macroscopic view will serve us in laying the foundations of our comprehensive model, but we will use a microscopic view when we are trying to illuminate those points that appear to be crucial as viewed from a distance, so we are seeking to verify details in a limited range.

The power of numerical models is obvious, but we also recognize that the application of the techniques of natural sciences to the social sciences, including the clinical arts, too often results in dealing only with those problems that are open to measurement, independent of their intrinsic import. By contrast, the aim in this work will be to deal with problems of importance independently of their susceptibility to measurement. After all, it would be foolish to try to deal only with those things for which the model provides a tight fit. Society appropriately expects that we will use our clinical skills in helping communicatively impaired persons now being neglected. In many cases we are not providing skills because there are no clinicians available, and we are currently experimenting with the use of "sub-professionals" to help bridge the gap. But we have concerns that do not stem from a shortage of clinicians. There are problems in evaluations and therapy, problems in teaching such techniques, and most significantly, problems in trying to bring the techniques and results of much modern intellectual and instrumental sophistication to bear on our clinical skills. In order to increase our effectiveness in all these areas, as well as to have "sub-professionals" assume a role in therapy, we must understand more fully the components of our own arts and crafts.

Any clinician who makes predictions is operating from some model, whether or not he can detail it to someone else. It must also be obvious that any two models giving comparable implications from clinical decisions are operating upon equivalent information and are equivalent rule structures. Therefore, no reasonably experienced and successful clinician should expect to be greatly surprised by what he finds in the following pages. There are no facts in the book that are not already comprehensively covered in the fundamental fact-synthesizing texts in the discipline.

All of us can ask of the model: Does it give my therapy direction? Does it enhance my evaluative approaches and techniques? Does it help me understand the implications of my clinical decisions? As long as the model supplies insights, it is useful. Further, as it supplies insights it also demonstrates that there are the kinds of commonalities in clinical processes that have been suggested. If this is so, we can examine the commonalities with a view toward refining our activities and undertaking our tasks with increased assurance.

This, then, is the fundamental orientation of the book. The human being will be viewed as a perceiver of complex information whose perceptions are to a great degree determined by what he expects to perceive. We have considered that no one can store everything he experiences, and that "labeled" material will be retained, though not exclusively so. This memory-stored material determines what will be perceived subsequently, in the sense that one tends to observe what he is prepared to observe. The role of this book in training the student is to make clear what kinds of information should prove most useful in serving his professional growth. The simple but general model will guide the clinician, practicing or prospective, in thinking about what kinds of things must be perceived in order to make competent clinical decisions of many varieties. The sections following the development of the model will deal both with applications of the model in various types of clinical encounters and with implications of the model for various professional activities, particularly in the areas of training and research.

TWO

The Model

Human knowledge might be looked at as a set of past decisions. We can as easily call this knowledge a set of immediate biases or, to say it in a somewhat less colored manner, a set of accepted hypotheses. All three ways of characterizing our internal state of knowledge mean the same thing. We are talking about what we know and how we view the world. "What we know" is one of two major divisions of our state of knowledge and can formally be considered as our data—our observations, perceptions, memories. "How we view the world" is the other major division of our internal state of knowledge and it can be considered formally as our set of rules for generating new hypotheses.

The two major divisions of our knowledge continually interact. Our sets of rules certainly determine in a large degree which new sensory impressions we will consider important enough to commit to memory and which will be forgotten. Alternatively, our success in dealing with the world should influence whether or not we alter our use of the rules. However, I profess no insight as to what the set of rules might be and therefore cannot discuss whether new knowledge could influence the rules we use (in other words, I am not prepared to discuss whether the rules are learned or can be systematically altered by learning). Mathematicians and engineers who deal with self-controlling mechanisms state that hypothesizing is a necessary condition for any automaton and they define hypothesizing as the manipulation of data according to an internal set of rules to reach decisions on future actions. A set of rules is necessarily built into any self-controlling machine and certainly the human being has a set or sets of rules "built in." The question is whether these rules are altered at all by experience. At least for the moment, my answer must be that I have insufficient data to reach a meaningful decision by any of the rules that I "know."

Preliminary Examples

THE MEDICAL CENTER

We find ourselves in a medical setting and more particularly in a Department of Otolaryngology. As we are aware, one segment of the clinical population finding its way to such a location is that relatively large group of persons who have laryngeal problems. Many of these problems seem to manifest themselves in vocal characteristics before the laryngologist can see any signs of tissue change, whereas others show tissue change before vocal accompaniments occur. In addition, as you know if you have ever experienced the evaluation regime of a medical department, a significant portion of those evaluated by such a clinic have no pathology ascertainable by either the laryngologist or the speech pathologist. We will examine the differing evaluations of patients by two persons, the laryngologist and the speech pathologist, and the evaluations examined will include some made of "normal" persons—those without ascertainable pathologies—randomly interspersed among the other two types of patients.

In the case of each patient, both clinicians must reach one of two decisions: normal or abnormal. Certainly there is always the exceptional case of a withheld judgment or a request for additional tests or consultation, but in the main, the patient is at the medical center for a process that requires this dichotomous judgment: normal/non-normal.

An examination of the decision process of each clinician would reveal it to be exceedingly complex. We will assume that there have already been established a rough set of ground rules indicating that the laryngologist will base his judgment on his examination of tissue color, tone, and the like, and the speech pathologist will base his judgment on criteria such as voice quality and pitch. In each case, the clinician goes through a process of evaluating his observations of this patient against a background of his memories of previous evaluations of normal persons and persons with pathologies of one sort or another. He takes *observational data* on this patient and pulls *comparison data from memory* on previous patients. He must arrive at some decision about where this patient fits into the vast array of patients he has seen in the past, because of the requirement of giving a dichotomous decision.

Speech pathologists might differ in some of the *kinds* of things they would listen for in the speech and voice of a given patient and, in addition, each might show some variability in the importance he assigns to each type of observation. But on the whole, there will probably be reasonably high agreement as to whether or not a particular patient is normal.

A number of laryngologists evaluating the same patient might differ in some of the criteria they use for their observations and might assign different values to their various observations in coming to individual decisions. But again there would probably be high agreement as to the decision for any one patient.

Because there are individual differences between the laryngologists or between the speech pathologists, we could spend a significant amount of time trying to compare the judgments made within either group. We could try to list all the things each clinician observed and evaluated, and whether most or all of the other clinicians used the same or differing observations; we could then try to discover the importance he attached to each item he evaluated relative to all the items on his list; and finally, we could consider whether the importance given an item in any list might have been influenced by his confidence in his own judgment.

From these explorations we could learn more about the individual making the judgment than we would about the pathology or the patient because gathering the three kinds of information for each examiner (the items on the list, the importance assigned to each item, and his confidence in each judgment) would reveal that each examiner gave us a somewhat different complex of knowledge.

Each would give us a different complex of knowledge precisely because each brings a different set of experiences to the examination. Let us for a moment examine the basis of such differences, because it is important and is a recurring theme. We have already noted that one's experience can be considered to be a set of accepted hypotheses, an internal state of knowledge or set of immediate biases that fall into two major divisions. The first of these comprises the basic data—one's memories of previous observations of other patients; the second major division constitutes the formal set of rules for generating future hypotheses. The rules decide what a person will place in his basic memory store and what he will choose not to notice and not to store. In addition, the rules determine what he will decide these new observations mean relative to past observations and past decisions—that is, the rules determine how he puts his information together.

Each of us is already familiar with the marked differences in perception found among different people in the same circumstance.

There are countless instances of eyewitnesses giving vastly different and often directly conflicting reports on the same sequence of events. Our previous delineation of the two divisions of knowledge illuminates how such disparate eyewitness reports can be generated. In many instances, witnesses have formal sets of data that are sufficiently different to cause them to pay attention to distinctly different portions of the set of ongoing events. Inevitably, then, different observers will leave the scene with different sets of data and different ideas about their meaning (different hypotheses derived from the data). Finally, they have different recall abilities in addressing memories from their own storage systems, and distortion creeps more or less significantly into the reports made by each observer.

Just so, each speech pathologist, or laryngologist in our example would give us a different knowledge complex because each brings a different set of experiences to the examination. If we are willing to grant, for the sake of our example, that most frequently they are correct in their clinical judgments, then obviously it is possible for different clinicians to look at the same patient in many different ways, and to gather different observations, assign different values to observations, or have different levels of confidence in their observations, and still all reach the proper decisions.

Admittedly, the rules for decision-making are not known, and so we cannot know definitely that everyone makes decisions in the same way. It is a fact, however, that we use different information to reach the same decisions. The implications of this are that there may be no single way—no optimal set of observations underlying a complex decision. Many sets of data may be used; in addition, no matter how long and hard an individual tries, he may not be able to tell us what he observed to get the data he used in making his decision, or how he used the data once received.

To the degree that any speech pathologist is a competent clinician, he can be expected to have sets of knowledge whose importance in making decisions is comparable to similar but not identical sets of other competent clinicians. These disparities occur because of the examiner's expectations about the examination rather than anything in the examination itself. Each clinician must examine various aspects of the patient's behavior and compare these observations with his memories about normal patients and patients with some pathology. Though we don't know the specific rules, we can say that the clinician must place his perceptions of the patient, which include his observations, the values he assigns to them, and his confidence in his judgments, on a scale combining the same kinds of judgments taken from memory so that he can come to the single decision: normal or pathological.

In a clinical decision, even though there are many factors that must be evaluated, we need concern ourselves with only the last decision: Is the patient normal or not? We can think of a single dimension, called the Decision Axis[1], along which the examiner places his knowledge-complex. This knowledge-complex underlying the decision axis may be exceedingly diverse both in nature and in internal relationships but finally it can be viewed as resulting in some single number magnitude representing the patient on the decision axis. The examiner evaluates this magnitude relative to his decision criteria in labeling the patient.

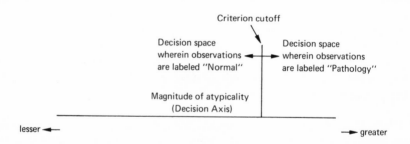

FIGURE 1.   *A decision space for evaluating the limits of normal functioning.*

The experienced clinician, therefore, has built into his professional intellectual equipment some location where he can make the direct comparison of the patient under current evalution with other patients, both normal and pathological, and rank order all of them. He can "see" if the patient falls into the normal group or the pathological group and label him as one or the other. Probably the clinician doesn't actually rank order the patient, but rather orders the magnitude of his deviance from some kind of average in persons labeled as normal. And, at some location sufficiently far from the average value of the normal group, he now places the label abnormal or pathological (see Figure 1).

To understand why a clinician takes a complicated variety of con-

---

[1] A series of abstract terms, of which Decision Axis is one, are introduced in the following pages with only contextual definitions, but are systematically defined and discussed beginning on page 24.

siderations and places them along a simple decision axis, consider the following question: How serious must a functional articulation problem be before it is worse than a moderate stuttering problem? Anyone who says that this question cannot be answered has never found himself in the position of being able to add only one more child to his caseload. We may not like such decisions and we may argue that they cannot legitimately be made, but we also find ourselves making them and discovering that it can be done. This kind of decision requires placing each patient on some type of decision axis by assigning a magnitude of need for assistance, and choosing the patient who falls farther along the scale.

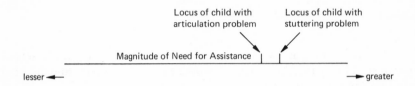

FIGURE 2. *A decision space for evaluating patients' needs for therapy.*

The operation of separating normal from abnormal will be described in a later section; for now, consider the clinical conference of the two examiners, the speech pathologist and the laryngologist.

These gentlemen must sit down together, reach a decision about each patient, and give the patient some feedback. They must say something is wrong, or nothing is wrong. In the former case they must prescribe some therapy, and in the latter case they must release the patient, perhaps with some discussion of his symptoms.

The easy way for our clinicians to start this fusion process is to eliminate from discussion those cases on which they agree, and then discuss patients about whom they disagree. Each examiner can put his patients into two classes and, for our two competent examiners, we would expect these classes to show agreement by holding the same people. For the examiners' decisions considered together, therefore, we will have a group of patients about whom there is agreement that they are normal, a second group about whom there is agreement that they are pathological, and two additional groups, representing each examiner's list of patients about whom he considers the other examiner in error. From whichever viewpoint we care to examine the interaction, we can say that the distribution of patients on the decision axis of the laryngologist does not show precisely the same rank ordering as the distribution of these same patients on the decision axis of the speech pathologist. Some patients on each side of each clinician's normal-abnormal "fence" are found on the other side of the other clinician's fence. Therefore, the joint clinical labeling behavior, considered from the point of view of either, gives us a four-way classification system of patients: X called X, Y called Y, X called Y, and Y called X.

We will leave our friends to resolve their differences in any way that serves their continuing mutual satisfaction and benefits their patients. We will return for reconsideration of some of the other issues that have been raised. At this time, we move to quite a different setting and a very different but most common problem.

THE PUBLIC SCHOOL

For this example, we will examine the role of the public school therapist. The system in which he works has had a speech and hearing program for a number of years, a state law fixes the maximum caseload, and the superintendent is accustomed to year-end reports indicating: a routine caseload heavily concentrated in the lower grades; a caseload of approximately 70 percent functional articulation problems; and dismissal of 40–50 percent of the caseload at the end of the year. (Later we might profitably discuss some of these criteria but for the moment let us accept them as representing the expectation of the superintendent.)

As you can see, this is the most typical role in the profession, and perhaps the most frustrating. But the elementary school clinician is the backbone of our profession and our model must be useful here if it is to have any lasting merit. Let us, therefore, take as an example the most common problem of the elementary school clinician.

Sometime early in the fall there is an appraisal of new students, which includes first graders and all transfer students of whatever elementary grade. A significant number of first graders cannot produce all sounds adequately in all positions with any consistency. However, not all these children with misarticulations are in need of therapy, though some of them may never achieve phonetic mastery without it.

How does the therapist decide which first grade children should be given therapy and which should not? He cannot take all of them because of caseload restrictions. He is reasonably ethical as a therapist and wants to spend his energies as profitably for the children as he can, though he is also aware that the superintendent expects almost one-half of the caseload to be dismissed by year's end.

What an examiner must do in this situation is to create two

groups which we can call "Future Articulatory Normal" and "Future Articulatory Defective." Then he can relase the first group back to the classroom and schedule the second for therapy. It seems reasonable to assume that there will be some children placed in the Future Articulatory Normal group who should not be there, and they will be revealed in time because they will not achieve the mastery of articulation that the examiner predicts. However, there are also probably some children placed mistakenly in the Future Articulatory Defective group, and the therapist will be unable to find them because they will achieve mastery of articulation skills and he will conclude, incorrectly, that this was the result of the therapy. Therefore, if he desires to be able to determine that he placed the children properly, he must give no therapy, return all children to the classroom, and wait. In later examination, he would be able to place them in four groups. Two groups will comprise those rightly said to be normal and those rightly said to be articulatory defectives. And of course the other two will be those thought to have fallen on one side of the fence but who ended up on the other side (see Figure 3).

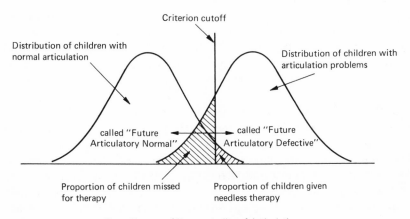

FIGURE 3. *Labeling behaviors as a consequence of establishing a criterion cutoff.*

We will have good reason to return to this second example because it is very much a real-life situation. It does not occur quite as we have stated above; instead, probably we go through something like the first labeling process and, in fact, schedule the Future Articulatory Defective group for therapy. But the fact that we make mistakes in this labeling (only a few, we hope) means that we do not give therapy to that portion of the group labeled Future Articulatory Normal who will in fact have articulation problems, but we do expend therapy time on the portion of the group labeled Future Articulatory Defective who would achieve phonetic mastery with no more than the passage of time. Some children do not get therapy they need while others get therapy they do not need. This is the public school dilemma to which we will return. For now, let us remind ourselves that both of our examples have the common characteristic of a four-way classification system: X called X, Y called Y, X called Y, and Y called X.

THE SPEECH AND HEARING CENTER

We require one further example that will carry us beyond our present common ground. Our hypothetical clinician now is the out-patient examiner in a speech and hearing center and he is presented with the following problem. A young lady of four years appears one day in the company of her parents, whose chief complaint is that she stutters. He evaluates the girl's speech in formal recitation and spontaneous conversation, with and without her parents (perhaps with each singly and then together), and in their company without his presence. He goes through numerous evaluative and interviewing techniques with the parents and child. The evaluation includes multitudinous components and the decision is complex. Let us, in our example, agree that the little one is normally dysfluent.

Why is this example like the previous two? There are not four categories, if for no other reason than there is only one patient to consider.

In all three examples we have the common factor of a complicated set of observations and perceptions, all of which must eventuate in a decision: normal/non-normal. In each case that decision came about because the decision axis contained a criterion cutoff—a fence—so that if a patient were perceived as falling on one side we considered her normal and if she fell on the other, we called her pathological.

The girl's parents, however, went through the same set of considerations and reached exactly the opposite conclusion. Why? Did they observe very different behavior? Presumably not, because the examiner systematically inquired into the girl's speech in other situations and took these parental perceptions into consideration in his decision. He obtained reports of their observations, made his own evaluations as to the confidence he placed in the parents as observers, and then assigned some magnitude of importance (weighting) to these considerations in reaching his decision about the girl's speech.

What alternative explanations are available? One obvious possibility is that the parents heard a few instances of dysfluency and assigned too high an importance to these isolated occurrences. Perhaps the parents have not heard or paid attention to normal dysfluencies of other four-year-old children, so while their perception of their daughter may be accurate, their perception of the appropriate criterion cutoff separating normal from non-normal is not reasonable (see Figure 4).

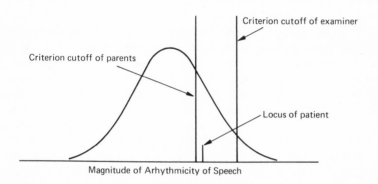

FIGURE 4. *Criterion placement (labeling behaviors) of parents and of examiner.*

An observation falling to the left of the criterion cutoff would be labeled normal; one falling to the right would be labeled stutterer.

Components of the Model

We now have enough common material in our examples to allow us to begin to consider the form and structure of our model. We know that each decision about a patient includes two perceptions. One is the patient's location on the decision axis and the other is the location of the cutoff. If this gradation is valid, then it is appropriate to consider the large number of clinical decisions that can be made on this simple decision axis. To this purpose, therefore, let us reexamine our examples and ask the question: What kinds of observations are located along the simple decision axis?

Our medical center speech pathologist must have a decision processor containing distributions (sets of memories) of a variety of attributes (such as voice quality) for persons of all sizes, shapes, and ages. He will have distributions of those characteristics as they are typically or atypically found in persons with normal voice, and distributions of those characteristics as they are found in persons with pathological voice. Obviously, the speech pathologist must have the former and it will be helpful, though possibly not necessary, that he have the latter (we will take up this issue in a later section).

His laryngological colleague has comparable sets of distributions not built on vocal quality but rather on tissue tone, color, and the like. In addition, he probably stores sets of distributions on broncho-esophageal phenomena, pharyngeal phenomena, and so forth, both for normal and pathological patients.

It is appropriate to consider that these two distributions—normals and abnormals—overlap. This is true precisely because even our simple decision axis is derived from such a complex set of phenomena. If we had an ideal clinician who knew precisely what should be observed in each patient, had complete confidence in each observation, and could render to each the exact importance it deserved in his set of observations, then he would have an ideal decision axis. Each person upon evaluation would be placed at the appropriate location in a rank ordering and the ideal clinician could, without error, label patients according to any set of characteristics he might choose to use. This would yield, by whatever set of characteristics, a distribution of persons along the decision axis who fell to the normal side of this ideal clinician's criterion cutoff and a distribution of persons who fell to the non-normal side. Because this ideal clinician could compensate for the day-to-day variability in his patients and their presenting symptomatology, he would show the same two distributions at any time and would be equally consistent in his labeling (his placement of the criterion cutoff). But human clinicians are not so omniscient in perceiving clinical signs nor so consistent in applying clinical labels. For these real observers, the complex interrelationships among these phenomena, observed with more or less confidence and given more or less importance in the decision, most certainly should be considered as giving birth to

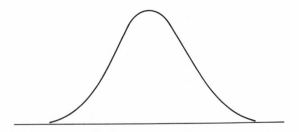

FIGURE 5.   *The normal distribution representing the occurrence of complex variables in large populations.*

a less than ideal decision axis, so some overlap of the two distributions can be expected to occur. This means that we can expect to find some "jitter" in any decision that is close to the cutoff. Perhaps seeing that same patient with the same set of symptoms on a different day would give rise to the other decision, but at this time they do not.

Because the distribution of the normal population, as expressed along the decision axis, would have in it so many variables, some independent and others interdependent, it would most likely be normal ("bell-shaped") in form, so we will represent the distribution by the normal distribution curve (see Figure 5).

When we intermix two decisions, as in our example, the situation becomes even more complicated. The individual decision axes will map onto one another with great effective similarity but they will not be congruent. Their joint distributions give rise to four classes of patients and, as we have already discussed this, we can move on to consider the distributional aspects of the second example.

The public school therapist with a group of first grade children represents a superficially different problem. We can consider the example as presented so that in September there is only a single population,

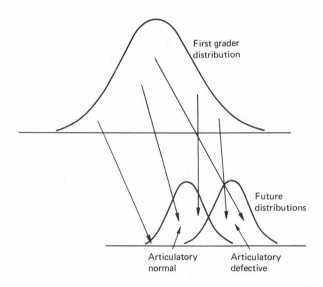

FIGURE 6. *The distributions of articulatory competence in children as first graders and as advanced students.*

whereas at some later date there is a distribution of articulatory normals and a distribution of articulatory defectives (see Figure 6). In fact, the September population appears to be a single one only because our techniques are not precise enough to allow sorting. The two underlying distributions: "Future Articulatory Normals" and "Future Articulatory Defectives" show significant overlap by presently measured characteristics.

Perhaps with more precise tests we will be able to sort these two groups out when they are early first graders. Some programs and clinicians seem to perform early sorting better than others, but with present methods, the two groups are intermixed and we cannot completely sort them at this time.

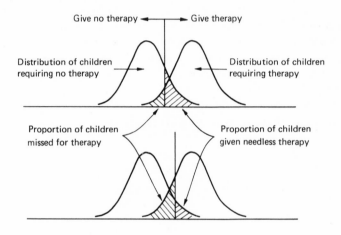

FIGURE 7. *Influence of a shift in criterion to reduce the amount of unneeded therapy.*

A First Potential Use of the Model

We should take a few moments to examine an aspect of this unfolding explanation. We have discussed the idea that there are two potentially mistreated groups of first grade children: those who require therapy they do not get and those who get therapy they do not need. The first group comes from the right-hand distribution (children requiring therapy) but falls to the left of the decision criterion cutoff as this fence is placed by the examiner; the second group comes from the left-hand distribution (children not requiring therapy) but falls to the right of the fence. Suppose we move our cutoff to reduce some of the useless therapy. This means, in our Figure 7, moving the fence (criterion cutoff) to the right. As you can see, the shift in criterion has the desired effect because a smaller proportion of the distribution of children is subjected to needless therapy by being labeled "Future Articulatory Defective." However, the same shift in criterion has the result that more of the children in the group requiring therapy will now be labeled "Future Normal" so that an even larger group of children than previously will now miss therapy they require.

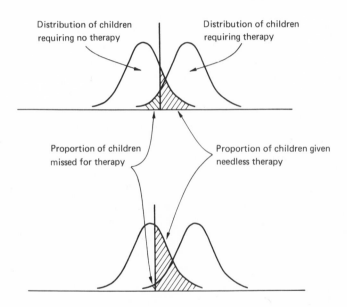

FIGURE 8. *Influence of a shift in criterion to reduce the number of children missed for therapy.*

"That's all wrong!", we say. We must move the fence the other way in order to give therapy to those children who do need it and are not getting it. Remember, moving the fence in this manner means becoming more willing to call any child a "Future Articulatory Defective" (see Figure 8). This increases the number of children who will be thought to need therapy and it will therefore have the desired result: children needing therapy but not getting it because they have been labeled "Future Articulatory Normal" will now be labeled "Future Articulatory Defective" and will receive therapy. But as we can see in Figure 8, this result can be accomplished only at the price of taking still more children into therapy who do not need it.[2]

Certainly, as one moves his criterion cutoff he will alter the relative amounts of X called X, Y called Y, X called Y, and Y called X. But he cannot alter only one without altering the other three. All four are fixed in relationship by the amount of overlap of the distributions on the decision axis, and a change in criterion cutoff to alter any one group alters all four.

The Intrinsic Structure

Now most of the structural components of our model are visible and we can examine some of their interrelationships in the abstract. Where it seems that an example will enhance understanding we will take time to consider one, but the three we have already presented should serve this function without any necessity to derive others.

We have referred several times to the concept that the decision axis is of simple construction with complex underpinnings. A decision axis represents some kind of dimension along which is scaled each of the perceiver's observation sets for a large number of observation sets. In our three examples, each observation set represented the complex group of determinations made on a single patient so that the result is a judgment point of greater or lesser magnitude along the scaled decision axis; that is, each observation set (each patient) is used to generate a single point.

We have used and defined two terms: observation set and decision axis. Both are fundamental to the skeleton of our model and we will discuss each in great detail in the next two sections. In discussing each term, we will introduce two applications: the first is a hypothetical ideal, and the second is the genuine observation set or decision axis such as we would find being used by a clinician. The distinction will be

---

[2] Momentarily going outside the framework of our model, there seem to be three ways out of this dilemma: (1) to find new tests that can do this early sorting with greater accuracy and reliability in order to reduce the overlap between the two distributions; (2) to hold off any therapy at all with first graders or even second graders, waiting until the children are old enough to be sorted out with the evaluative techniques that we do have; (3) to utilize therapy techniques so much more efficient than those we currently employ that the cost of putting all these marginal children into therapy will be low enough to make this an economical solution to the mislabeling problem. Nonetheless, as long as the groups show their present distributional relationship, alteration in location of the cutoff (becoming more willing to make a particular decision) has implications for all four classes of response.

quite clear so that there will be no question as to whether the ideal or actual is under consideration, and you will see the reasons for both applications as we proceed.

OBSERVATION SETS

We can profitably begin our discussion of observation sets by using an analogy to develop the distinction between the ideal and the actual. I will place before you a movie screen displaying a table with thirty-nine objects on it. The objects are familiar to you and I will ask you to study them carefully because you will be asked to list as many as you can from memory. To aid you in the task I will pay you a thousand dollars for each one you list. Unfortunately, I will display the table for only ten seconds.

How well do you suppose you will do? Unless your memory is exceptionally good, you won't do as well as a camera worth less than twenty dollars because it can "recall" all the objects from a ten-second scan. You might recall about seven. Perhaps your visual memory is quite good, and we will allow that your motivation might be high, and you may do even twice that well. You would, in this latter case, be doing about a third as well as the camera.

If we suppose, further, that I am observing along with you and have about as good a memory and equally high motivation, I might also be able to recall about fourteen. But we would expect that many, if not all, of the fourteen I recall would be different from those you recall. If we recall different items, don't we have a situation much like the differing observation sets of several speech pathologists? Presumably your experience would predispose you to attach more importance to some of the items than to others and probably these higher-valued objects would be the ones successfully recalled. Presumably, I would do the same but for some or all different items.

We can label the set of objects you recall your *observation set,* and we should be reminded that the label includes the observation itself plus the importance assigned to it by the observer (you) plus the influence of your confidence in your own observation. I have, in the same situation, my own observation set. We are already aware that the observations in the two sets are at least partially different and so we have good reason to believe that the observation sets differ even more. And, finally, we have the picture taken by the camera, which might be considered our ideal observation set; the camera values all objects equally and has absolute confidence in its own observation accuracy in that it does not question or downgrade it.

In order that you not dismiss the example as trivial, let us put it into perspective by considering a more realistic clinical concern. We could return to any of the three examples which introduced the model, and we will arbitrarily use the example of the school clinician. The clinician evaluates children in the fall of the year in order to choose a caseload. There are many children for whom he is responsible so he can spend little time evaluating each one. Typically he will reach a decision about including or excluding a child by sampling some small set of the total spectrum of behaviors of the child. The child seen on Monday who was awake watching television very late Sunday evening may present a very different sample of behavior than she will if seen Tuesday, after falling asleep early Monday evening. If we suggest that the clinician watched the same late Sunday television show and also fell asleep early Monday evening, clearly we would have sharply different observation sets generated Monday and Tuesday.

The physician ordering an additional laboratory test that many of his fellow physicians think unnecessary is operationally expressing his desire for a more comprehensive observation set. The elderly bachelor lady who checks the locks on her windows and doors three times before retiring is operationally expressing her confidence in her observational powers with respect to the importance of the observation for her observation set.

What would we consider the ideal observation set for the young lady being evaluated Monday or Tuesday? The collection of every behavioral trait that could give insight into her speech, hearing, or language performance, when observed as fully as necessary to allow complete confidence in the observation, and when considered in the full light of all the other components of her behavior, would make up the ideal observation set.

An ideal observation set is a theoretical limit—an absolute ceiling on any possible actual observation set. It is all the characteristics that could possibly be used by any observer to shed light on the observation. What may not be so obvious is that the ideal observation set is defined in the absence of any concern about human observers; it depends solely upon the characteristics of the patient. All the characteristics of the ideal observation set on the patient have some potential importance even though some examiner or all examiners are without sufficient insight or skill to notice many of these characteristics. If the patient alters in her speech, hearing, or language competencies, so would the ideal observation set on her.

Our discussion has dealt with two actual observation sets on the patient as well as the ideal and we have agreed, for hypothetical purposes, that these sets are probably quite unlike one another. Further, we should expect that somewhat different observation sets would be generated by evaluating the same patient on several successive days. In spite of all this variability, we tend to arrive at essentially identical conclusions about the patient, whether we consider different evaluations by the same examiner or examinations by different examiners.

So we begin to appreciate the complexity underlying the concept of an observation set. The observer is a clinician who must render some clinical judgment. He will do this by observing among a relatively small group of behaviors of the patient. Some of these behaviors will be rigidly structured by the clinician, other behaviors will be more or less controlled by the examination milieu, and still others will be relatively freely determined. The examiner knows that much of this behavior is redundant but he cannot predict the time-course of occurrence of successive bits of nonredundant behavior. He needs as large a selection of this restricted sample as he can get in order to maximize the contents of his observation set, so he must be ever watchful (and that is an exceedingly energy-consuming task). Further, the examiner knows that some observed phenomena are more important than others for his decision, so that a part of the inferential process subsequent to observing each atom of behavior is the assignment of a weight reflecting its importance. Additionally, if the clinician is wise, he also assigns some sort of confidence rating to the observation, reflecting his willingness to believe his observations. All these considerations are in our definition of an observation set— observation plus weighting plus confidence judgment.

Why should we arrive at essentially the same conclusions with different observation sets? Might it be because our conclusions are so gross that we can ignore wide variations in the information needed to reach the conclusions? I think not. Rather I think that reaching the same conclusion from various observation sets suggests that the underlying process is ergodic in nature; that is, the perceptions that different clinicians have of the patient converge even though different observations are used in sampling the patient's behavior. Processes having statistical characteristics such that sampling at different times yields converging descriptions are called ergodic processes. To say that the human being can be so described means that he engages in persistent patterns of behavior and also that different persons observing him at different times can reach the same conclusions about him.

We seem to be concluding that while one can formulate an ideal observation set, there is no single actual observation set that can be considered necessary to reaching conclusions about a patient. For each different kind of observation set there may be a minimum amount of input appropriate to a reliable decision, but what an appropriate minimum might be would vary from observation set to observation set. The specific elements included in each observation set would also vary.

In later chapters we will have cause to return repeatedly to the concept of individual differences in observation sets. It would be comforting to our early training anxieties if there were only a single set of observations appropriate to any decision on any particular patient. If this were so, we could learn how one determines what the set must be for each patient and then insure that each of us learned how to obtain the set when he had determined its constituents. One of the great problems in becoming clinically competent is that there are different ways to "skin the cat," and while we may feel that one observation set is better than another, the aim in early clinical activity is not to learn what is the best observation set (if, indeed, there is one) but rather to learn some adequate set. We could, should we desire, derive a type of efficiency measure for the person generating an observation set by comparing his set with that of the ideal. We indicated above that such a measure would not necessarily be appropriate for early clinical exposure, although such a measure, if we could arrive at a reliable one, might well provide a way of evaluating a clinician with respect to certification of competence.

Answering the question of what an adequate set is requires discussing goals for establishing particular kinds of observation sets and is not immediately appropriate. We will deal with it when we consider the use of the model in clinical service; our present concern is establishing the structure of the model itself.

DECISION AXES AND DECISION VARIABLES

The discussion about observation sets has dealt with the knowledge that must be gained from a patient if reasonable decisions about some aspects of his communication problem are to be made. The public school clinician must make a dichotomous decision: normal/therapy prospect. In the example of the speech and hearing center examiner, the decision was to be normally dysfluent/stuttering. In these examples or in any other, we have an observation set on a (prospective) patient that we must compare with observation sets, pulled from memory, of other patients and of persons having many of the same observed behavioral traits but considered to be normal.

The substance of the observation set is evaluated through the assignment of a sort of index number called a decision variable, and the decision variable is located along a dimension called the decision axis. Each observation set results in a single magnitude placed along the scaled decision axis. For each additional person we observe we generate an additional magnitude of the decision variable so that, with sufficient numbers of observations, we would gradually develop distributions along the decision axis. One such distribution would represent persons considered normal in whatever characteristics we have noted in our observation sets. But we are clinicians and presumably we will also develop a distribution or distributions of persons having some speech, hearing, or language problem.

For some kinds of communication problems the elements of the observation set may be of such a variety that the range of the decision variable for the distribution of persons considered normal does not at all overlap the range of the decision variable for the distribution of persons considered as non-normal. The occurrence of a cleft of the palate may, on the average, provide such an example. But even for this example, many persons can be found whose voice quality seems very like that of persons with submucous palatal clefts, and this type of cleft may be found for some of the group but not for others. Any decision axis using a variable strongly determined by nasal voice quality might show the distribution for normals somewhat overlapping the distribution for persons with clefts. The decisions we reach about any individual arise by evaluating the location of his decision variable on the decision axis and answering for ourselves the question as to whether the magnitude is more like what one would expect if the observation set reflected the characteristics of the one distribution or the other (or a third, fourth, and so forth) —in this case a distribution of persons with nasal voice quality but normal palatal structure or a distribution of persons with nasal voice quality associated with palatal clefts. We know that we will err in our observation sets and in our judgments so that our judgment also will reflect our greater willingness to make one kind of labeling error rather than the other.

Of course, the choice of components and the weights and confidence ratings assigned to them will determine how much overlap there might be for a distribution of normal persons and a distribution of persons with some pathology. Many times our goal in clinical research is to find some measure or measures that will help to differentiate these two distributions and to increase their separation on some new decision axis. In a like manner, one of the indications of growing competence in clinical skills is a growing sensitivity to the subtle and not-so-subtle cues that a master clinician uses to generate a decision axis on which a normal and a clinically pathological group have as great a separation as current technology will allow us to achieve.

We have implied that changing any aspect of an observation set— its observations, the applied weights or the confidence ratings they receive —would result in a different decision variable. A systematic change in these components of a decision variable for the observation sets newly observed or drawn from memory results in a new decision axis. Changing any particular component in each observation set would result in a different index number being derived for the observation set and might result in differences in the locations of the observation sets in a distribution. Obviously, if the change results in all the observation sets in each distribution shifting by a constant amount, effectively nothing will have changed. If the change results in all the observation sets of only one distribution shifting by a constant amount (see Figure 14), then the distributions will be closer together (and have more overlap) or farther apart (and have less overlap) than previously.

We expect that the component observations in an observation set occur in different amounts in different persons so that altering the occurrence, weight, or confidence of a single component probably alters the value of many observation sets differentially, and alters the locations of many persons in a distribution relative to one another. If this more likely situation occurs, so that altering the structure of an observation set shifts the people in the distribution around, then it is appropriate to say that the new distribution occurs on a new decision axis.

The clinician using different elements in his observation set employs a different decision axis than you do. It may be that his use of these different observation sets is such that the locus of any point on his axis bears the same relation to all other points as the locus of that point bears to all other points on your decision axis; that is, the process is ergodic. In that case you and he would have on your decision axes the same distributions even though you derived them using somewhat different observation sets, which is probably what happens with experienced clinicians. It seems reasonable, as a first approximation, that they have about the same distributions on their decision axes, though these were probably derived through somewhat different observation sets.

For our illustrative grade-school therapist, we might consider that there is a hypothetical decision axis along which are distributed the children as they *will be* when they achieve mastery of their phonetic articulation as far as they are going to do so without therapy. We talked of this dimension previously, asserting that the children fell into two groups, and we labeled them as "Future Articulatory Normal" and "Future Articulatory Defective." When the children are evaluated in September, a genuine decision axis (reflecting present perceptions) is constructed, employing whatever techniques might be useful—the future decision axis is approached as closely as possible. To the extent that the September decision axis differs from the future decision axis, there will be four classes of students: X labeled X; Y labeled Y; X labeled Y; and, Y labeled X—the same four classes under discussion previously (see Figure 9).

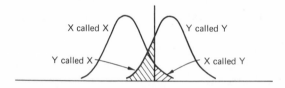

FIGURE 9. *Generalized labeling resulting from establishing a criterion cutoff.*

In addition to considering the structure of a decision axis and the distribution of points (observation sets) along it by assignment of greater or lesser magnitude of some highly complexly derived composite measure (decision variable) to each person evaluated, presently or in the past, we should spend some time examining the *criterion* by which an evaluator decides that a person belongs in group X or group Y. We will require, first, only a very short tangent to point out that there is no reason why a decision axis need be restricted to only two distributions. One could, for example, construct a decision axis on some characteristics such as hair color and there would be a range from deep blue-black, through brown to red, to blonde, and finally to white. One could also place a series of criteria to contain, within their borders, only those with deep brown hair, or blondes excluding redheads, and so forth. This example should both bring home the realization that there can be as many criteria on a decision axis as one desires to make decisions, and simultaneously, it should make obvious that the criterion, like beauty, is in the mind of the perceiver.

Of course in the clinical interaction, our concern is not with anything nearly as simple as hair color. Rather we reach decisions about questions like: Does this child have a learning disability? Should that adult aphasic be considered for an intensive therapy program? Will this child profit more from a residential school for the deaf or from a combination of private therapy-tutoring and a normal high school?

Each of these can be considered as requiring a decision axis with a large number of distinct observation sets, every bit of data evaluated and weighted and the entire group somehow squeezed into the derived measure (decision variable) we assign to our evaluation of each patient. One might disagree with the concept that a decision axis should be a single dimension, such as height or color. Many of us might consider the attempt to squeeze diverse data onto a single scale as a gross over-simplification of a complex multidimensional process. The concept of a simple single dimension follows from the kind of decision that the decision axis is used to evaluate. Simply stated, one must compare the patient with an internalized normal and decide that the patient is or is not within the normal range. If nothing but the age of the patient is changed, we may be forced to consider an entirely different concept of normal, but we are forced nevertheless to reach the same kind of decision: normal or non-normal. (An example of this is an evaluation of the voice quality of an eight-year-old as against an eighty-year-old male.)

If we alter any aspect of the observation set, we may have to consider the patient with respect to an altered decision axis; but the decision remains one of evaluating the complex of factors as seen in the patient, and the same complex of factors as seen in a wide variety of other people, previously observed and previously labeled. Ultimately, we find ourselves comparing the patient's magnitude of characteristics and deciding that it is sufficiently great and he has pathology or it is less great and he does not. As long as this is the important operation, it seems that we can agree to consider it as occurring on a single-dimensioned decision axis.

THE CRITERION CUTOFF

We introduced the significant considerations in the establishment of any criterion cutoff when we discussed what happens if one shifts his criterion in labeling first graders. When we consider that the distribution of persons along a decision axis is not going to be, on the average, the same as the distribution of persons on the decision axis we would *ideally* construct, then we must be prepared to deal with these two classes of mislabeled people: normal labeled non-normal, and non-normal labeled normal, as well as with the two classes of correctly identified persons. We saw that if a criterion placement is strongly determined by the desire not to waste therapy, the fence will be so placed that few children are labeled as needing therapy and getting it who, in reality, do not require it. That is, the size of the group labeled "Future Articulatory Defective" is reduced and thereby so is some of our marginal mislabeling (fewer normals are labeled non-normal). However, we also thereby increase the size of the group labeled "Future Articulatory Normal," increasing the number of marginal mislabelings (non-normals labeled normal) and increasing the number of children not getting therapy they require.

If, on the other hand, we are willing to expend therapy needlessly on some children in order not to miss those children who require therapy but might not receive it, then we move our criterion cutoff the other way with the alternative joint result. Increase the size of one group, including those incorrectly labeled as belonging to that group, and thereby decrease the size of the other group, including those incorrectly assigned to it also. And, very simply, we do so by considering the advantages and disadvantages of each kind of decision and each kind of error. Each criterion cutoff location leads to a decision involving less error of one type at the cost of more error of the other type, so "you pay your money and you take your choice."

The most appropriate way to define a criterion is to consider it the ensemble (collection) of locations on the decision axis leading to the same decision. Any observation set magnitude leading to a particular decision is *in the criterion* of that decision so that one shifts criterion when he reaches a different decision. This definition of criterion, while perhaps initially strange, is fundamental, whereas the other terms, fence and cutoff, do not hold the ensemble property of a criterion but serve only to limit a distribution at one end.

Our future considerations of criteria will concentrate heavily upon the relative values and costs of increasing either type of error in order to reduce the alternative error. We should remember, however, that when we relocate any criterion cutoff we alter the labeling for all four categories and not only our mislabeling behavior. If, for example, we reduce the proportion of normals improperly labeled non-normal, we are increasing the proportion of normals correctly labeled. And we have already pointed out that when we move the criterion fence to alter our labeling behavior in the manner described above, we also decrease the proportion of non-normals labeled correctly and simultaneously increase the number of non-normals incorrectly labeled as normal.

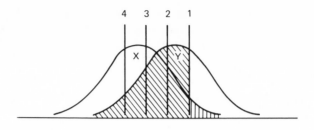

FIGURE 10A. *Locations of four arbitrary criterion cutoffs.*

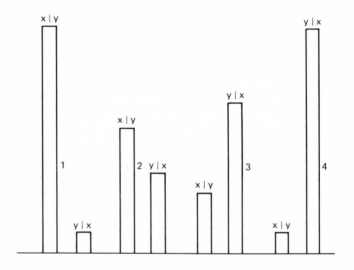

FIGURE 10B. *Relation of proportions of two types of labeling errors for the criterion cutoffs shown in figure 10A.*

The proportion of observations drawn from distribution Y and labeled as being from distribution X because it fell to the left of, for example, criterion cutoff 1, appears in 10A as oblique shadowing, and is labeled in 10B as X/Y (read: called X, given Y). The proportion of observations from distribution X labeled Y because it fell to the right of criterion cutoff 1 is shown in 10A with vertical shading and labeled in 10B as Y/X (read: called Y, given X).

THE PAYOFF MATRIX

Statistical decision theorists, who expend great energy in consideration of results of various kinds of decision, talk about advantages and disadvantages using a slightly different vocabulary. They call advantages values, and disadvantages costs, and they call the consideration of values and costs involved in a decision a *payoff matrix,* sometimes abbreviated as payoff.

A complete discussion of the utility of a payoff matrix in statistical decision theory is well beyond the scope of our consideration and also beyond our present need. Many books can be found that will introduce any interested reader to the mathematics of incorporating values and costs in his own decision processes.[3] We will dabble in payoff only to the extent of sensitizing the reader to the role it plays in guiding the user to an optimal decision behavior for any specified goal structure. At the same time we alert the reader to two points: (1) decision theory does allow construction of an optimal decision criterion, and (2) the optimum demands a prior establishment of one's goals. Altering the goal structure may result in a different optimum.

Let us suggest the flavor of the influence of whatever strategy might be used to optimize the behavior of some clinician. We will temporarily deviate from all clinical concerns and enter the familiar area of everyday money management.

One kind of decision maker might employ a *minimax* strategy— *he minimizes the maximum risk.* This person might be very willing to place a two dollar bet at a race track early in the month in the hope of increasing his moderate supply of money. He will not do so toward the end of the month (just before payday) because if he loses the bet he goes without dinner. A better example might be the man who continues to drive, though he is very aware of the accident statistics and some of the inherent engineering faults of modern mass-produced vehicles, but his minimax strategy results in his wearing his shoulder belt every time he is in the car.

Another observer might employ a *maximax* strategy—*he tries to maximize the maximum gain.* This man might go without lunch for a week to buy three Irish Sweepstakes tickets. He does not care that his likelihood of winning is so astronomically small that buying three instead of one scarcely begins to bring the probability of winning anywhere into a reasonable range. He only thinks of how much he will win if he does win.

[3] One of the most readable presentations I have found is in a paperback entitled *Design for Decision* by Irwin D. J. Bross (New York: The Free Press, 1953). For a presentation of decision models and decision making in the human being, with particular attention to the experimental results, see *Decision Making,* Ward Edwards and Amos Tversky, eds. (Baltimore: Penguin Books, 1967).

To contrast our two observers, let us suppose that each has a business with a working capital of $10,000 and each is offered the possibility of investing all $10,000 in a fast deal that will double his money though he stands a one-in-four risk of losing it all. On the other hand, each can invest his $10,000 in some salable items for the business that will, without question, net him a $1,000 profit. We do the mathematics necessary to consideration of this example by saying that the expectation for the first deal is:

$$(\$10,000 \times 0.75) + (-\$10,000 \times 0.25) = \$5,000.$$

The first part is the probability of success (0.75) times the gain $(+\%10,000)$, and the second part is the probability of failure (0.25) times the cost, if failure $(-\$10,000)$.

The expectation for the second deal is:

$$(+\$1,000 \times 1.0) = \$1,000.$$

The 1.0 is the probability of success and there is no considered probability of failure, though one could for sake of completeness add to the equation the following term $(-\$10,000 \times 0.0)$.

The first deal is, on the average, five times as good as the second deal and the maximax observer will take it. The minimax observer will refuse to consider it because one thing not in the equation is the fact that if the deal fails, not only would he lose his $10,000 but he would also lose his business from lack of working capital.[4]

Actually one could also place this business risk into the equation as long as he is willing to assign a dollar value to what it means to him to lose his business. As a matter of fact, like the little boy who does not want to go to the store to earn a dime because he already has a dime, one can even use units other than money so that the units have equal value. After all, the boy is only saying that the second dime is less valuable than the first, and the businessman who uses the minimax strategy can be considered as saying that the $10,000 working capital has a greater value, dollar for dollar, than the $10,000 possible gain (or the $5,000 expectation, to be more precise).

One of the more potentially insightful aspects of the use of a payoff matrix is the necessity for each value and each cost in the decision to be examined and assigned some magnitude or weight (a value being a

[4] This particular example is adapted from I. D. J. Bross, *Design for Decision*, New York, Free Press, 1953, pp. 112-13.

positive weight and a cost a negative weight) Further, the magnitude to be assigned, and perhaps whether it is to be a value or a cost, is determined by the goal system of the decision maker. If his goals change, then he may assign different values and costs than he did previously so that he may reach a different decision even though he considers the same features on both occasions.

There are different strategies that can be used, of which we suggested only two: a minimax and a maximax. Further dimensions become important when one is evaluating repeated decisions of the same variety by any decision maker attempting to optimize his behavior. Most of these additional factors deal with how one alters the definition of optimum as one alters the elements in the decision being optimized. We are developing a model for application to clinical problems and it is not germane to deal with behavior of a decision maker in repeated samplings. It is somewhat more difficult to deal with the question of strategies, because different clinical problems call for different strategies, so this topic is best left to a later section.

What placement of a criterion cutoff means, practically, is that one must assess for himself what it will cost if he tends to make an error by calling a normal client non-normal, as opposed to what it will cost to make an error by calling a non-normal person normal.

Of course, one may not realize what that cost is, but presumably this is part of what one learns in training for a profession in speech or hearing. The parents of the little stutterer paid the cost of labeling her in order to get the value of expert assistance. One who believes in a diagnosogenic theory of stuttering etiology would shudder to think what cost that labeling might have demanded of the young girl in later years, had the label remained. This was a cost attached to the payoff matrix that was not in the perception of the parents, though the clinician may consider it to be wise counseling to put it there.

In the case of the first graders, the cost of moving the fence one way or the other has already been indicated, though the previous discussions have passed over several questions. What does it cost the child if we hold off therapy for functional articulation disorders until the phonetic inventory is fully developed? Is therapy more or less effective, and more or less efficient, in first or in third grade? Is it better to let a child with a functional articulation disorder or a child with a harsh voice wait for therapy until the next year? What does it cost to handle more difficult cases so that only 20 percent of the case load is dismissed by the end of the year instead of 45 percent? What will it mean to my working relationships with the laryngologists if I insist that there is a potential pathology in a patient's throat, and a biopsy, which the laryngologist thinks unnecessary, shows me to be wrong? Suppose it shows me to be right? Should I label the girl a potential stutterer so we can get the parent(s) into counseling and relieve some of their stringent goals for her? All these questions are significant in establishing criteria because they do influence our judgment; that is to say, they are already in the matrix that will determine my criterion so that it may be merely wisdom to become aware of that fact and try to bring them into a more systematic consideration.

What is an Optimal Criterion?

If it is true, as has been suggested, that establishing a criterion for clinical decisions involves such a variety of conflicting value judgments, how can one reach an optimal decision? I believe the answer rests in the term "optimal decision" and is definitional. When the clinician evaluates the things he considers important to the decision, evaluates the relative importance of each, and then puts them together in a manner analogous to the profit considerations described in the previous example, he is in a position to determine where to place his fence with respect to the magnitude of the complex quantity (decision variable) his patient must show before he will be called X rather than Y.

Unfortunately, most of these considerations are outside the range of this model or any model because one is asking for a way to objectify judgments about issues that are social questions. Whether one decides to give therapy to too many children in order not to miss those of marginal mislabeling or, conversely, rejects a selection of children for therapy because some would get it needlessly, is going to be determined by the psychosocial attitudes of the judge, not by his clinical competence.

What is important is that while such considerations are outside the framework of any model, there are procedures for helping reduce the uncertainty of such judgments, because judgments must be made whether we feel competent to do so or not. One such procedure for reducing their uncertainty might involve, as an example, assigning money value (or some other utility unit value) to each of the costs and values involved in each kind of decision and tallying up a balance sheet. While this procedure is a superficial approach, it does have the marked advantage of making us aware of exactly what variables were or were not considered in our decision and also what we consider to be the relative importance of each.

There are, of course, decision axes one constructs for decision processes in speech and hearing where a criterion does not involve such dramatic and difficult choices. For example, we are all aware that what we call a phoneme is a distribution on a series of phonetic features bounded by criterion cutoffs. If we distort (and we will discuss the criteria that underlie the decision 'distort' in just a moment) particular characteristics of the /s/ phoneme sufficiently, we will have a "slushy" /s/ which, if we continue to increase the magnitude of distortion, becomes an /ʃ/. If we agree that this is possible and even a common occurrence, we are agreeing that there is a decision axis with a distribution on it we label /s/, another distribution that we label /ʃ/, and a cutoff placed somewhere between them. There are many variations on the target phoneme /s/ that we might consider atypical or distorted but that we nevertheless will agree belong in the phoneme. There are other distortions we will not accept as being in the phoneme; these fall into the /ʃ/ phoneme though they are probably also distorted productions of that phoneme (see Figure 11).

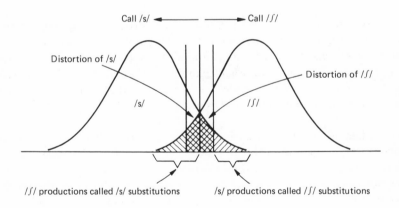

FIGURE 11. *The influence of criterion cutoffs on substitution and distortion labeling behavior.*

This seems to support the idea that a deviation from the normal or typical allophonic production of /s/ serves to define a criterion, and that there are greater and greater distortions of /s/ as the production deviates more and more from the norm, until the magnitude is such that we consider it a different distribution and label it now also a distortion, but a distortion of /ʃ/. If the word in which it appears requires an /s/, the phoneme is a substitution; and the greater the distortion on /s/, the lesser on /ʃ/, except that at some arbitrary location we change the label.

In general, we can agree as to whether a production is an /s/ or an /ʃ/, though there will be cases of clear ambiguity wherein one makes quite an arbitrary decision. Most of the time the linguistic context is so compelling that it need be no problem, though one can construct examples in which the misunderstanding might well make a significant difference. Typically not, and we do not fuss about the matter, because a small shift in criterion in either direction makes no important difference.

The criterion problem is one of the most difficult for the professional and, I believe, insights toward resolving it will come directly from accumulated clinical wisdom. However, there are some sociological considerations in the matter, and these are examined in the chapter on research.

The Model as a Structure

By now we have looked at the entire structure that will be used in the remainder of the discussion. In order to pick it out of the particulars of presentation, we will discuss the ideas concerning the structure that we have used in one or another example so that we can talk about the inherent variables of the model itself. Specific applications in therapy, evaluation, and in training and research will follow.

The basis for the model is a decision axis considered to be a simple single-dimensioned intellectual space. We assert it to be single-dimensioned because it serves as the location for decisions made through consideration of some magnitude of a decision variable, even though the decision variable may be highly complex in the number and kinds of observations of which it is composed. It may be helpful to repeat that the decision axis does not necessarily have to be single-dimensioned; it can be any number of dimensions. We could, for example, describe a chandelier as being a certain distance on the dimension from floor to ceiling, a certain distance from a side wall and a certain distance from the back wall. Alternatively, we could project all three dimensions onto a string from one wall to an opposite wall, so placed that it goes through the location of the light fixture. The chandelier then could be located by giving only one observational value of the distance from the wall. Either is a complete description of the point at which the chandelier is located and our argument would be the same by whatever frame of reference better satisfies any particular reader. We have chosen to conceptualize the model in a single dimensioned space rather than a multidimensioned space, but either would be satisfactory.

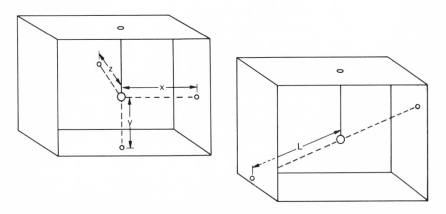

FIGURE 12. *Locating an object in finite space by specifying three dimensions or one.*

On this axis one acquires observation-set points so that he gradually builds one or more overlapping distributions. The concept that these points form distributions is, at its heart, a decision—the axis simply contains a large number of points.[5] But we can say with some comfort that

[5] Throughout this section of the discussion is the implicit and pervasive construct of the "ideal" set of distributions; that is, the normal and non-normal distributions we would generate if we labeled people by use of ideal perception. The construct is purely hypothetical—useful, but unreal.

The assertion of ideal sets of distributions implies that the perceiver "knows" what perceptions are important to the construction of his decision axis as well as the relative importance of each perception. In short, ideal axes and sets of distributions deal with the knowledge the perceiver can bring to bear, whereas typical axes and sets of distributions deal with the knowledge he *does* bring to bear. In the process of employing these perceptions optimally, he constructs an ideal decision axis and distributes his patients along it. One large group of these observations will fall into a distribution centered on the magnitude of the very complex quality (which underlies the decision axis) that represents average normal, and another large group of such observations will fall into a distribution centered on the magnitude of the quality that represents average pathology. We build decision axes and classify people—quite arbitrarily —as belonging to one distribution or another because doing so helps us organize our world. And in like manner, we can construct a hypothetical ideal decision axis, as we have done. But this construct remains only hypothetical, and people

human beings are economical in their accomplishment of repeated intellectual tasks so anyone would tend gradually to group his observations, which is what we mean by the formation of distributions. In the area of clinical decisions, we have already said that these sets of observations have very complex underpinnings. They are made up of a significant number of details, many of which are going to be independent of one another. We would expect, therefore, that the distributions would tend toward bell-shaped (probabilistically "normal") and also that they would not actually terminate at either end. For example, we expect for most people that tongue size is about the same in proportion to oral cavity size. We also know that it would be grotesque for a person's tongue to be disproportionately small or large, though in a world of more than three billion people there may be a child born without a tongue or with a tongue occupying essentially the entire oral cavity. Whether or not we could find a child with either tongue condition would depend, to a large degree, how we defined a tongue or defined filling the oral cavity. Of course, tongue sizes would be expected to have some reasonable average, whether we fixed it either in absolute volume or proportion of oral cavity, and we would expect this value to be the one most frequently occurring. Higher or lower values would occur progressively less frequently as one moved away from the modal (most frequently occurring) value. We expect this result because we believe that there are probably many independent factors affecting tongue size and, for any given person, some factors would work toward a result greater than average and others would work toward a result less than average, so they would tend to cancel out and result in an average measurement.

This is characteristic where any complex of factors, commonly independent of one another, acts to determine a single result; its distribution throughout a population tends toward normal, which is what we would expect to find for the distributions on our decision axis.

If it is the case that many independent factors go into the location

---

do not *fall* into distributions on the basis of any criteria; we *place* them in distributions which we construct for our own purposes. There is no such dichotomy as normal people and non-normal people—there are just people. However, let us not draw the conclusion that the construct of an ideal dimension is a straw man. We will return to the point later, establish its importance, and try to do justice to it when we consider implications of the model for training. But all decision axes are bases of judgment, and the distribution of observation sets found on any decision axis arises from judgments. There is no perceiver-independent "objective" set of distributions for deriving judgment magnitudes about things as complex as any clinical matters we are likely to consider.

of any single point on a decision axis, why should there be more than a single distribution? The answer to this requires a simple restatement of the previous notion. If there can be considered to be some magnitude of a property that represents the degree to which it is normally present, then those persons showing a pathology would do so by adding (or subtracting) some variable amount of that property—as such change is what leads us to define the state as pathologic. In a large number of persons with pathological conditions, we can expect to find some average increment, added to (or subtracted from) each normal value. This would result, for a large number of pathologically afflicted persons, in a distribution much like the normal in shape but moved to the left or right by the average amount of the increment or decrement from the pathology (see Figure 13).

Let us take our discussion even a bit farther. An individual subject will show some magnitude (of what we might consider as the expected

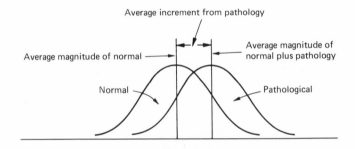

FIGURE 13.   *The influence of pathology incrementing some decision variable above normal magnitude.*

contribution of the property) which, for example, might be greater than average, to which might be added a greater than average contribution from the pathology. Another person might show us the same normal base to which is added only some small amount from pathology. These two people obviously would not retain their same relation in the pathological population as we have conceptualized them as having in the normal population. But these same influences acting on a large number of persons, some with a basic magnitude of the property and others with an additional magnitude of contribution from pathology, would result in a normal distribution and a pathological distribution, with about the same shapes; but the pathological distribution average would be displaced from the normal average by the amount of the average contribution from pathology.

Over time, one derives a large number of observations of persons with an absence of pathology; so large a number that the addition of any new observation would have no significant influence on the distribution, which would gradually assume a stable spread (variance) and mean location. We expect to find few observations considered normal that would deviate markedly from this mean, but we do expect that there will be some. In this sense, the distribution can be said not to have an end point. If there is an adjacent distribution, also without an end point, that we wish to keep separated from this one, we can do so only by choosing some end point arbitrarily. Out to this arbitrary point we can call all observations X, but beyond this point we will call them all Y, because it is more economical for us to store memories in such fashion. So we pick some location and use this to fix the range of our distribution. We have talked about such locations, and called them fences or cutoffs. We may now also think of them as being arbitrary end points of distributions.

Manipulating the Model

Two additional concepts should be understood about the distributions on the decision axis, which may have been obscured by the particular examples that have been developed. Distributions along a decision axis might represent such a thing as the productions of some phonemes by a single talker in conversations during a month's time. If we were unhappy with the precision of his articulation, there is no reason why we should not design therapy to move one distribution relative to the other—to alter its average value in order to improve their distinctiveness (see Figure 14). Alternatively, one might decide to keep each phoneme production distribution at its present value but alter the variance (spread) of the distributions so that all productions of each phoneme are more alike than they were before (see Figure 15). In other words, two avenues open for manipulation of a distribution on a decision axis are altering its mean or its variance, and we shall consider representative examples suggesting when each is a good therapeutical strategy. Either approach leads to increased distinctiveness between distributions but often only one of the two is potentially available to a patient so that the strategies of using either approach should be part of the armamentarium of the clinician.

Changing either or both the mean location of a distribution or its spread relative to another distribution alters the relationship of the four derived classes we have mentioned several times before. If we have two distributions with some criterion cutoff and we move the right distribu-

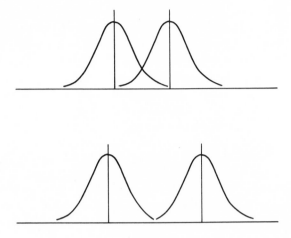

FIGURE 14. *Increasing distinctiveness by altering means.*

tion still more to the right without changing the fence's location, we will continue to mislabel as many observations from distribution X as being Y's, but we will label fewer Ys as being Xs, and more Ys as being Ys.

Instead of continuing to discuss distributions in terms of Xs and Ys, let us recast our terminology. Let us assert that whatever our distributions may represent in observation sets, our interest focuses upon the right-

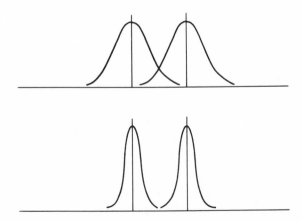

FIGURE 15. *Increasing distinctiveness by altering variances.*

hand distribution. All members of this distribution correctly labeled we shall call "hits." All the members of the same distribution incorrectly labeled as being in the left-hand distribution, because they fall to the left side of the criterion cutoff, we shall call "misses" (see Figure 16).

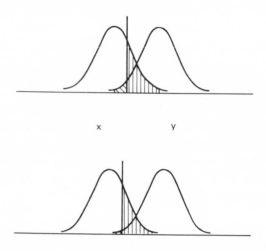

FIGURE 16. *Effect of increasing distributional distinctiveness while holding a constant criterion cutoff location for left-hand distribution (constant false alarm proportion).*

If a HIT is an observation drawn from the Y distribution and labeled as a Y, then a MISS is an observation drawn from Y labeled as an X, and a FALSE ALARM is an observation drawn from the X distribution and labeled as a Y.

The left-hand distribution also is split into two classes by the criterion cutoff. The members to the left of the fence are called "correct rejections." Those of the left-hand distribution to the right of the fence are "false alarms."

In Figure 16, we called the left hand distribution X and the other Y. Following our example, we focus our concern on the Y distribution. All members of that distribution correctly labeled, we call "hits" (Ys called Y), and those incorrectly labeled are our "misses" (Ys called X), and the entire distribution clearly is split by the criterion cutoff into these two classes. If we know the proportion of either, we can locate the placement of the fence on the distribution. In like manner, the same criterion cutoff split the total X distribution into "correct rejections" and "false alarms," and the proportion of one defines the proportion of the other and reveals the location of the fence.

If we move the distribution on the right still more to the right (increase its mean) without altering its variance or our criterion location, the false alarm rate remains the same, as this is determined by our left-

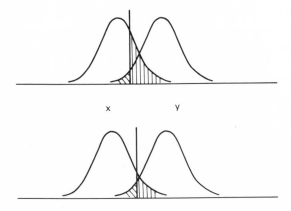

FIGURE 17. *Effect of increasing distributional distinctiveness while holding a constant criterion cutoff location for right-hand distribution (constant hit proportion).*

If a HIT is an observation drawn from the Y distribution and labeled as a Y, then a MISS is an observation drawn from Y labeled as an X, and a FALSE ALARM is an observation drawn from the X distribution and labeled as a Y.

hand distribution and the fence, but the hit rate rises as this is determined by the right-hand distribution and our criterion (see Figure 16).

If we had displaced the right-hand distribution and moved our criterion the same amount at the same time, then we would have kept the same hit rate and diminished our false alarm rate (see Figure 17). Note that the first (displacing the mean of Y without changing cutoff) reduces errors of omission (misses) but holds the same rate of errors of commission (false alarms); whereas the second strategy holds errors of ommission constant but reduces errors of commission. A moment's reflection may make us realize that, in general, society prefers the latter. It is much less antisocial to let a man drown because we do not help him than it is to help him to drown—one typically requires an explanation as to why we did not help, the other wins us a murder trial.

In Figure 13 and its accompanying explanation, we were dealing with the separation of a pair of distributions, where the left-hand one was of a population of persons normal in some manner, but the right-hand distribution was of a population of persons showing pathology by use of the same observation set. In such a pair of distributions, we derive some proportion of hits and some proportion of false alarms for any location of criterion cutoff we choose to use.[6] If we chose to move our criterion to the left and thereby to label correctly a greater proportion of the right-hand distribution as having pathology, we also inevitably mislabel more normal persons as having pathology. In our new terminology, an increase in hits is accompanied by an increase in false alarms. They vary together though at different and varying rates (see Figure 10 for this same point, expressed in terms of the two types of labeling errors that result).

If we assume a distribution representing some decision variable as found in normal persons and consider pathological occurrence of the decision variable to be an atypical magnitude (that is, some normal amount plus some increment), we achieve a certain overlap between our two distributions. The magnitude of the overlap would be altered by any change in the spread of the distributions or their average values. But for any particular pair of distributions, with whatever means and variances, there will be a fixed relation between them. Changing the location of a criterion cut will alter both the hit and false alarm proportions, but it will not alter the relation existing between the distributions. Therefore, whether the criterion of a specific clinician were rigorous (allowing few false alarms but, therefore, few hits) or lax (resulting in many hits but many false alarms), the relation of hits to false alarms is determined by the location of the criterion cutoff and the distributions. How we place a criterion will determine how we divide one population into hits and misses, and at the same time, how this means we split the other into false alarms and correct rejections. If we move to increase hits, we must be prepared to deal with increased false alarms; and if we move to decrease false alarms, we inevitably settle for fewer hits.

The figures used in the text display the mutual dependency of the hit and false alarm proportions by use of normal distributions but the form of the distribution is not necessary to the model and the only claim made for a normal distribution is that of intuition. A different form of distribution might yield a different hit-false alarm relationship. It is important only to appreciate that whatever the form of the distributions might be, there will be some hit-false alarm relationship (a curve relating

---

[6] You may note that we must specify either a "false alarm" proportion or a "correct rejection" proportion, because either is 1.0 minus the other; and we must specify either a "hit" proportion or a "miss" proportion. It is conventional, though arbitrary, to deal with "hits" and "false alarms," as both are observations called Y.

hits to false alarms, see Figure 21) that is independent of the criterion chosen by the observer. His criterion cut will represent a point on the curve relating hits to false alarms but the curve is determined by the distributions and their distinctiveness (the difference in mean value relative to the variance), not by the choice of any particular criterion.

Two final points on our model. First, the placement of a criterion is a highly complex and individual matter. Presumably, one of the things that one learns in training is to place a criterion with finesse and to have it vary only minimally. But if I happen to be a bit more lenient than you so I choose a criterion allowing somewhat more "sloppiness" in normal speech than does yours, there may be significant implications for some children: therapy or nontherapy; medical referral; alerting parents and creating anxiety in some about their child's speech, and the like. Notice, however, that this conclusion is not necessarily based on my having a different idea than you have about the occurrence, the magnitude, the degree, the range, or any other aspect of pathological or normal populations. It need only be on my locating my decision fence differently.

An additional implication that should not be overlooked is that anyone's perceptions of these distributions and their degree of overlap need not resemble these same distributions as they occur in the real world (that is, as we would collectively consider them). As a matter of fact, not only need internal distributions not agree with those of the world, there need be no internal agreement in sets of what are typically considered complementary distributions.

To highlight this, let us consider the case of a youngster who says /fin/ for /sin/. The child with this problem has a different set of internal distributions for generating these sounds than we have. His speech generation distributions are different from our generation distributions and, of course, from our reception distributions. In our extreme case, his problem may be that he does not have two generation distributions but only one. Further, there is evidence suggesting that his generation distributions may differ from his own reception distributions because he may hear the difference in the signals delivered to him from the speech of others, and perhaps even in his own correct productions that are recorded and reproduced to him at a later time. If, in this latter case, he does not hear the difference in his own immediate productions, it should suggest that in evaluating his own productions he uses immediate feedback primarily on the motor production side rather than the auditory reception side, and/or his distributions of sound productions take precedence over his distributions of sound receptions when both are invoked.[7]

If one reminds himself that a distribution of sound productions represents the population of some sorts of memories for speech generation patterns and a distribution of sound receptions represents the memory for auditory receptions of many productions of this sound by many persons over a long time, the problem may be that the child has not reached the stage at which he ties these two distributions together and keeps each in check by comparing it with the other. The issue will not be resolved in this section, and may not be resolved to the satisfaction of the reader at all, but the reader should remind himself of the *kinds* of things we are discussing even though we may seem to be using terms without much psychological referent.

These examples and clinical considerations are to remind us that we are modeling clinical processes—decision processes—and we must not lose sight of the fact that we are dealing with processes channeled through some perceptual mechanisms. We are concerned with decisions founded on sets of complex observations as stored by faulty memories which take in perceptions filtered by our vast experiences and our expectations of the world around us. While most of us look at the same world, there is very little reason to believe we all see it in the same detail. If our gross perceptions do not agree, some of us may be in serious mental trouble, but clinical processes are more concerned with fine detail than gross perception, and our appropriate concern with fine grain generates both our realization of individual differences and our consideration of a model structuring the features we hold in common.

Let us see if we can summarize our modeling of a structure we use or can use for decisions of clinical importance in speech and hearing. The basis of the structure is some location in our nervous systems, some intellectual space, where we can think of ourselves as bringing together the knowledge (observation set) we have about a person of potential clinical interest. This location has been called a decision axis and can be thought of as a kind of ruler—a scaled single dimension. The knowledge about a patient that is delivered to this decision axis is compressed into some magnitude of a variable, obviously quite complex, called the decision variable; and the components that must be compressed into the decision variable include our observations of behaviors, unstructured or

---

[7] For further discussion, see R. L. Milisen, "Articulatory Problems," in *Speech Pathology*, R. W. Rieber and R. S. Brubaker, eds. (Amsterdam: North-Holland Publishing Co., 1966).

structured (as sets), weighed by our perceptions of the relative importance of the several observations and by our confidence in the quality of the respective observations.

These components of our observation set (observation, confidence, and importance) yield some magnitude of our decision variable and are plotted as a point on the decision axis. Additionally, we pull from memory a large number of other magnitudes of our decision variable, each one indexing the location of some other patient seen in the past and stored in memory as a set of perceptions of the same type (observation set). If our observations have been insightful, the location of the points representing the large number of patients will tend to cluster into two or more distinct groups, each approximately bell-shaped. These groups will have some average separation but because the decision variable is complex in its components, because we do err somewhat in making observations, assigning confidences to our judgments, and inferring their value to our observation set, there will be more or less overlap (running together) of adjacent distributions.

Human beings tend to store memories by named groupings—by perceived categories—so labeling is an early (and, most often, necessary) process preliminary to some action. The more complex a phenomenon under observation, probably the more complex the structure of the observation set and the more categories we may finally arrive at (and the smaller the membership of each). Determining in which of n categories an observation set should be located involves comparing the magnitude of the decision variable associated with it and the magnitudes of the averages of the several categories, considering the values and costs of making each of the several possible decisions (that is, deciding where to locate our decision criterion cutoffs on the decision axis) and arriving at a decision.

An improper choice of decision axis (not considering some components necessary to the decision, too heavily weighting some components, or the like) must lead to an improper decision; a poor choice of criterion cutoff might lead to a poor decision. Repeated decisions on the same decision axis involve the types of labeling errors discussed earlier, and the poorer our discrimination, the more errors we will make. Changing the location of a criterion cutoff may or may not reduce overall error but it does alter the particular mix of errors that occur. Increasing discrimination reduces error, and which kinds of errors will be reduced is a joint product of the discrimination and the location(s) of the criterion cutoff(s).

Analysis of clinical behaviors has, at its heart, sequences of clinical decisions. These decisions may pertain to labeling processes called evaluation and diagnosis, they may relate to therapy goal planning and therapy strategies, they may relate to training students to some level (criterion) of clinical competence, or training supervisors, or sub-professionals, and a wide variety of other tasks. Many of these decisions are, much of the time, clear and straightforward; but many others are difficult to make and difficult to justify to ourselves or others, because the external facts seem so like some other set of facts where we seemed to have reached an opposite decision. It is the purpose of the model to display the skeleton of the decision process because the same decision process will be shown to underlie the greatest portion of this wide variety of clinical decisions.

Successive chapters will show the same decision model repeatedly put to use in dimensions of clinical concern: evaluation in both speech areas and hearing areas, therapeutic considerations in both areas, research needs in many aspects of the profession, and training considerations brought into focus by our decision model. Each of these areas is discussed, partly because of the intrinsic merit of the discussion but also and primarily as a continuing set of examples of the power of the model qua model.

In using the model we will vary our focus, sometimes concentrating upon the clinical interaction of patient and clinician, sometimes upon the behaviors of one more exclusively. But if we are to enhance our insights into these processes while we estimate the contribution of our model, we must consider them for what they are. They are decisions and the acting out of decisions, some quite consciously planned, others arrived at and executed with little deliberation. If the model is useful and insightful, one of the gains we will make in using it will be a greater internal consistency in our clinical decisions and actions, and a sharper focus on the goals of those decisions and actions. So let us begin a systematic application of the model into one area of major decision making—the clinical evaluation.

THREE

Clinical Evaluation Processes

Evaluation in speech and hearing, as distinct from therapeutic processes, is a domain of significant interest. In the area of audiology one need only evaluate university training programs, or salary schedules for various positions in audiology, or research reports on audiologic subjects, to realize that work progresses in audiologic evaluation almost to the exclusion of any area of rehabilitation (except, perhaps, hearing-aid fitting).

The same emphasis on labeling rather than remedying appears to be in the offing for speech and language pathologies. Certainly, there appears to be higher status attached to being a pathologist or diagnostician than to being a mere therapist.

It is easy to offer a variety of partial explanations for the seemingly higher status given the evaluator than that accruing to the therapist. Perhaps there is some merit in the assertion that pinning a label (that is, locating the patient relative to a fence separating normal and pathological) is more difficult and requires greater training than bringing that same patient to the permanent change in behavior that represents adequate communication. As we will see, the tasks of evaluation and therapy are so different in most cases that the question of which requires more training is of little interest and is perhaps unanswerable. But it does seem clear at this time that we reward evaluation and evaluators with higher status than therapy and therapists.

A reward system differentially treating labelers and therapists is particularly puzzling when we stop to consider that the diagnostic labels we use tend to have little inherent value. If we know an individual is a moderate stutterer, a mild dysarthric, or an early otosclerotic, have we delineated a therapy strategy or even a therapy direction? Indeed not! We require much more knowledge of the patient to be able to detail directions, goals, and tactics for therapy. As a matter of fact, we could gather all the other insights needed to embark on a successful or potentially successful therapy course, and probably realize that little if any contribution is made by the label. Categorization schemes based on general diagnostic labels appear to persist in spite of their very limited utility for the therapist. Their longevity suggests they have high utility for someone, however, so let us consider why.

Teaching speech and hearing has been oriented toward diagnostic labels for at least half the life of the discipline, and certainly much of the research into clinical phenomena is structured economically by use of diagnostic labels. The keeping of records, even therapy records, can perhaps be done most economically by use of diagnostic labels. Surely, statistics of various types for use by the profession might be less clear were any alternative labeling scheme used. But all these reasons are oriented from the focus of the clinician and not from that of the patient.

We could concern ourselves with the question of whether it profits the patient to be characterized by a diagnostic label, but we will not do so in a direct manner. Instead, we will ask a more general and more fundamental question: Who profits by the evaluative process which, almost incidentally, terminates in the labeling process? There is a fundamental sense in which the evaluation process need not be, but may be, of use to the patient directly. In order to examine this peculiar stance, it is necessary that we start with a set of ideas or assertions about patients in therapy.

We should have some initial understanding about terms, so let us begin with definitions of evaluation and therapy. An *evaluation* situation is one in which the information flow is structured to go from patient to clinician, and a *therapy* situation is one in which the information flow is structured to go from clinician to patient. Without question, it is almost impossible to consider a face to face interpersonal situation that does not involve bidirectional flow of information, but the definitions involve the concept of the intentions of the situations, even though they are contaminated in any real-world situation.

PATIENTS IN THERAPY

A patient comes for therapy because, somehow, he was motivated to place himself in the hands of a therapist for his speech or hearing problem(s). We can use the same terminology to deal with the patient (typically a child) who is in therapy because someone else brought him there, though the absence of an internal motivation may alter therapeutic strategies quite significantly.

The assertion that an individual is in therapy because something motivates him to come to therapy may appear so simplistic as to be idiotic, but it implies a great deal. It implies that:

1. If a clinician alters the patient's perceptions about his speech or about the conditions motivating his appearance at the S&HC, he may disappear without any alteration of his speech behavior, per se.

2. Any time during therapy that a clinician alters the patient's perceptions of his speech enough (and shortly we will talk to the point of how much is enough), he may disappear from therapy—drop out—independently of the objective state of his speech problem.

3. If a therapist discharges the patient before or after therapy *without* altering his perception of his speech, though the clinician may be quite satisfied about the adequacy of his patient's speech behavior, the patient will not be satisfied, and may begin to 'shop' for therapy but, in any event, he will be dissatisfied with the adequacy of the therapist and consider his therapy experiences less than successful.

4. Finally, and to the point on which we started, the patient perceives himself as having a problem and he comes to a speech and hearing therapist to remedy his problem. If the clinician requires an evaluation in order to start the process of therapy, the patient will probably put up with the evaluation. But he is not there to be examined—rather, he is there to be cured. He is in therapy to be relieved of whatever force motivated his seeking help.

We can recast the general idea into a form that squeezes it into our newly constructed model. The patient perceives himself as being at some location on a decision axis. His decision criterion cutoff was so located, relative to the value of the decision variable associated with him, that his decision was "seek no therapy." Something (unknown to us) altered his observation set and the magnitude of his decision variable with the result that he moved across the fence. Perhaps some additional information caused him to move the fence so that *it* crossed him. Our concern is not whether he moved or the fence moved but that he is now in the criterion space of a new decision—"seek therapy."

Someone or something in the environment caused a change in the decision of the patient so that he moved toward therapy. It may have been the sudden acquisition of some money, or a rebuff in a business or social situation which he perceives, rightly or wrongly, as being motivated by his speech. It may have been a professional recommendation. Whatever the direct cause, he was not in contact with a speech and hearing clinician previously and he now is; presumably to remain so until something new motivates him to terminate therapy.

The clinician must go through a variety of decisions prior to beginning therapy, and he requires an information flow from the patient to form the basis for these decisions. However, while the patient may realize that the clinician must go through such a decision process before personalized therapy can begin, the time spent in evaluation represents some variable delay between the time the patient schedules his first appointment and the time he begins to get some professional assistance.

We detailed four points, all of which hold significant implications for the evaluation process and, as we shall see, serve to structure the reasons for a clinician's evaluation. The argument, as it is unfolded, circumscribes the knowledge the examiner requires in order to do what the clinician wants—to engage in effective therapy; in order to do what the patient wants—to lose his necessity for continuing in therapy. This assertion is simply the other side of the argument made in number four above. If something provides enough motivation to change the patient's decision from resisting therapy to seeking it, then therapy will cease when anything occurs that reverses the decision.

Content of an Evaluation

In terms of the above discussion, two questions should be asked: What knowledge must be gained from the patient so that the examiner will be able to make use of the motivating force(s) bringing him to therapy in order to alter his communication behavior? What knowledge must be gained from the patient to keep him from leaving therapy prior to achieving reasonable goals, and then assist him in leaving therapy when he has achieved such goals?

Five varieties of information are necessary to a comprehensive evaluation of any patient. The first of these, which precedes the evaluation, is the estimate the clinician has internalized of normal speech, hearing, and language behavior. No estimate of deviance in communication behavior can have validity if the clinician does not have an excellent perception both of typical normal behavior and typical variance in normal behavior. Second, the clinician will derive some estimate of the magnitude and focus of the problems manifested by the patient. What is the patient's position relative to normal communication patterning?

Both of these components are recognized as appropriate to evaluation and are routinely manifested in evaluative procedures and the reports of clinical evaluations.

The additional items are less often represented in reports of clinical evaluations, though they are hardly less important. The first of these, a third portion of evaluation, is some prediction of the patient's potential performance. Unquestionably, predicting future terminal behaviors of patients is difficult and will involve errors both of under- and overpredicting (a later section addresses the topic of errors and their relative values and costs. See the early paragraphs of Chapter 4.) But the clinician can plan reasonable goals for a patient and prepare the patient for termination of therapy only if he can estimate and communicate to the patient the appropriate terminal behaviors to be expected. There may be many clients for whom the terminal behaviors at the time of discharge will be different from and less than the patient's ultimate communication behavior. The important point in therapy is that when the patient is discharged, his understanding, performance, and motivation are such that his communication will *continue* to be maintained or improved and he will have reasonable goals for his current and future performance.

We have already discussed the patient's perception of his own speech and his perception of the evaluation of others, in addition to concerning ourselves with an objective evaluation of his speech. This suggests that the clinician's appraisal of the patient's own perception of his speech is of importance, as well as some estimate of the patient's perception of *normal* speech. How aberrant does he consider his own speech and how atypical is his conception of 'normal' speech? These pieces of information form a portion of our estimate of the factors influencing the behavior of the patient. These factors, the values and the costs associated with various courses of action, delineate the motivations of the patient so that the clinician can fuse activities designed to accomplish reasonable speech goals (as the clinician, not the patient, would define them) with behaviors the patient will engage in because he views them as moving him toward terminating therapy. Hopefully, the patient will accomplish the goals set by the clinician—adequate speech performance—at the same time he accomplishes the goal he sets for himself—terminating therapy.

The final division of information consists of insight into the dyadic variables that can be expected to influence clinical interactions during therapy. It may be that the evaluator will not serve as the therapist, in which case the therapist will have to complete this portion of the appraisal during his initial interactions with the patient, but each therapist can be expected to use the motivations of the patient somewhat differently in his clinical transactions and must arm himself with insights into the interpersonal variables that will help to determine the changes the patient should undergo in therapy.

The evaluation, then, requires that five areas of knowledge be secured:

1. the clinician's evaluation of normal speech;
2. the clinician's evaluation of the patient's speech relative to normal;
3. some prediction of the final success of the patient, and the appropriate terminal clinical behaviors at the time of discharge;
4. the components of the patient's perceptions, including his perception of normal speech and his perception of his own speech relative to this normal, which will bring him to speech therapy and keep him there as long as necessary;
5. some insights into dyadic variables that will strongly influence the quality of the therapeutic interaction.

Probably many clinicians find themselves more or less in disagreement with the contention that these five informational areas are required. Some will argue for a different number; others will argue for different items. It does not seem worthwhile to argue against the possible assertion that identifying information is necessary, though one could reasonably state that while it undoubtedly helps the clinician keep his records and identify his patient, it makes no contribution to therapy, per se.

A clinician might also assert that there must be a comprehensive appraisal of the anatomy and physiology of the speech mechanism. His argument could be expected to propose that construction of reasonable goals and procedures for the therapy has such an appraisal as some requisite portion, as a necessary aspect of predicting therapy success.

Probably the argument has validity and it is probably true that the more insightful the clinician, the more the goals and tactics of therapy will be influenced by particularities of anatomy and physiology. However, except in very gross terms, there are no well-established relationships between anatomical and physiological variables and the variables influencing listener judgments of talker adequacy. Certainly, for many speakers with clefts of the palate, there is an associated nasal vocal quality and imprecision of plosive articulation. For many speakers who are missing incisors, there is also an associated imprecision of articulation of some of the frontal consonants. But not for all, in either case.

As we stated above, it is probably the insightful clinician who can make a reasonable prediction about the patient's expected performance in the face of some anatomic or physiologic idiosyncracy. But for many clinicians dealing with patients showing such signs we need a great deal of research before we can assert with any comfort the relations between a talker's anatomy and physiology and his speech adequacy.

Let us hold off argument as to whether an anatomical and physiological evaluation of the patient is a necessary preliminary to planning therapy. Also we will delay any consideration of whether current evaluation techniques are so organized that these five components are routinely obtained (we might be more accurate if we assume the examiner enters every evaluation with an appropriate distribution on normal speech and thereby requires acquisition only of the other four) or of how evaluations could be structured so that the components would be obtained. What is important is to appreciate that acquisition of all five kinds of knowledge, and perhaps more, is the goal of a successful evaluation.

Before dealing with any specific components of evaluation, we should try to speak to two points skipped over while presenting this introduction to speech-evaluation processes. There was, first, an early assertion that an evaluation need not be of any use to a patient, and there was, second, an early question raised as to how much a patient's speech can be altered before he will drop out of therapy.

The first of these involves the contention that evaluation does the patient no *direct* good and, as it typically is conducted, may do him little or no indirect good. The definition of an evaluative process as distinguished from therapy carries in it the implication that the evaluation is of no direct benefit to the patient: The only way this conclusion is invalid is if one argues that the patient will get information even from the questions he is asked and the tasks he must perform. Of course usually the patient will draw conclusions about what he is being asked to do. But what the patient derives may be of dubious value unless he happens fortuitously to strike upon an interpretation that is both correct and useful. What is directly beneficial to the patient is alteration of his speech, or alteration of his perceptions about his own speech adequacy in the event that his speech is adequate but he does not think it so. Both are derived from the information flow from examiner to patient, so they are not elements of evaluation, but of therapy.

To say that the evaluation may not even be of *indirect* value is to assert that too frequently evaluations gather insights of the fourth type— an appraisal of the patient's speech from the point of view of the clinician—and include data about the normal process but do not contribute toward the other types necessary. Two of the additional three aspects of clinical insight deal with the patient's perceptions and motivations; and not structuring the evaluation to obtain such perceptions and motivations asserts that they are not necessary to therapy. If these additional areas of insight are necessary, therapy will have only fortuitous value until they are obtained, if at all, and in this sense evaluation is said to be of no indirect value because they are unfinished at the time we typically conclude them. (The point is most important and we shall return to it.)

The second point requiring some exploration is the question of how much the patient's perception of his own speech can be altered before he might drop out of therapy even before reasonable goals have been attained. Obviously, the question is open to no simple answer, but is integrally related to the values and costs the patient assigns to remaining in therapy versus terminating therapy. For some patients, an offhand reassurance during the initial interview that the problem is not very serious may be sufficient to assure that the patient never returns; for others, therapy may meet so many needs that the clinician finds he is unable to get the patient to accept termination long after any reasonable speech goals have been achieved. This is precisely why it would seem that one must ask questions about the patient's motivations—his matrix of values and costs about his own speech behavior and his motivations, self-perceived or not, for being in therapy.

Questions about the patient's motivations are, by far, some of the stickiest to come to grips with, so rather than delay these considerations, let us try to deal with them now.

EVALUATION OF MOTIVATION

We begin with two questions central to evaluating a person's motivations: Can one predict another's behavior or even his own? If so, how is the prediction determined?

Our answer to these questions derives from behavioral psychology and asserts that one cannot deal with other than the observable behavior of another person. From such behavior one can infer such things as motives, ideals, goals, and philosophies of the actor, but all of these inferences are only probabilistically related to the individual under observation, because they represent decisions of the perceiver. These decisions have a greater or lesser probability of being correct depending upon the insight, experience, and observational powers of the perceiver. They represent the environment as it is sensed by all the modalities of the perceiver in combination with the multitudinous decisions about these sensory inputs that the perceiver makes, based upon his past experiences, his present expectations (predictions), and like considerations.

The outside world is important and we do expect it to be rational and predictable, and when it is not, the first thing to be determined is whether the "breakdown" is in the environment or in ourselves. For most people, we predict a relatively simple and straightforward relation between behavior and motivation. That is to say, we expect a man's behavior to be predictable from the combination of our observations and our rules for generating predictions based on those observations. We perceive another's actions in varied situations, we assume that his perceptions tend to be much like our own (though let us always be human enough to allow him to be somewhat more complex than he may appear!), and we reach some conclusions about how he might act in particular situations. (We will pursue, in a later section, the implications deriving from the idea that the perceptions of problem speakers—for example, the stutterer—can be assumed or shown to be different from those persons without similar problems.)

Occasionally we suspect a man is devious. We tend to find some disparity between what we perceive his motivations to be (inferred from our observations) and the actions we expect to result from such motivations. Shakespeare painted magnificent word portraits of many such persons, and a reading of history offers portrayals of many more.

The world around us offers, in addition, many persons whose motivations we feel we may not understand completely but whose actions we find admirable and consistent; and we consider such persons complex though we do not typically call them devious. We tend to find their motivations quite admirable if a bit too self-demanding.

In the everyday world, therefore, we all tend to feel we understand the relation between motivation and behavior and we do, in practice, consider the reaction to be a relatively simple one for most people. We certainly tend to operate in this manner though we also, perhaps, tend to disagree with the statement of the position until we stop to consider our own typical behavior. Patently the answer to the question of whether one can predict behavior of himself and of others must be Yes, or the world around us would be complete chaos. With most people, at least those under the influence of a Western European culture, in most instances the world seems quite regular and predictable.

This last thought probably holds the key to the question dealing with the components and procedures involved in the process of prediction. If we say the world is orderly with respect to our own behavior and the behavior of others, we are saying that we acknowledge some reasonable (predictable) set of behaviors that we expect ourselves and others to display in each of the daily situations in which we typically find our-selves.[1] We situationally define a decision axis and use some aspects of the appearing distributions as a base for prediction. Because this is true, one might ask further if exact predictions typically are made or can be made correctly, and to this question the answer, probably, must be No. We do not, and probably cannot, make exact predictions about the be-havior of others in typical activities. But we can discuss the general range of behaviors within which we expect the person to perform and, probably, the better we know him the narrower is the range of prediction.

How is the prediction determined?

The basis for predicting the behavior of others or of ourselves arises from our past experiences with—our distributions of memories about—the behavior of many people in what we perceive as being com-parable or analogous situations. Note that at least two components of prediction are a set of experiences of our own or of observations of the behavior of others, and a perception that the situation for which we make a prediction will be like some situation we remember. To say that one situation will be like another is to say that the components of the situation which will control the behavior of the subject are going to be very similar to the components of the remembered situations which con-trolled the behavior of the subject at that time.

In other words, we build a model to predict behavior. We define what we perceive as the controlling variables for the future behavior, sample from our own memories the behavior we have observed from persons like this person, and predict a behavior falling within the same range. And is this not the same type of process that we have been dis-cussing from the very beginning of the book? We are drawing hypotheses about behavior, and thereby asserting that we understand the underlying motivations, even though we do not know the rules that govern the process.

If our perception of the situation is not similar, in important detail, with that of the subject, then our prediction may not be very

[1] Irving Goffman, *The Presentation of Self in Everyday Life* (Garden City: Doubleday Anchor Books, 1959), presents an interesting discussion of the neces-sary collusion of actor(s) and audience in most social interactions which, if true, speaks directly to the abilities of all participants to predict the (limits on) available behaviors. A less interdependent interpersonal orientation is found in Carl Rogers, *On Becoming a Person* (Boston: Houghton-Mifflin, 1961), esp. Chap. 6, "What it Means to Become a Person." Rogers implies that situational predictability might routinely be reasonable because of the humaneness of the participants, but it is less assured.

accurate. If either we or the subject have had little or no experience with previous situations that had comparable controlling components, then our prediction may not be accurate. If the subject reacts differently to a situation than have other persons, so that the behavior we predict is not behavior that should be expected from him, our prediction may not be accurate. Each of these conditions of inadequate prediction of behavior arises from a failure in some component of a fourfold scheme:

1. the actor's (subject's) prediction of a situation;
2. his actual reaction to the situation (his behavior);
3. the predictor's perception of the situation, including the actor;
4. his prediction of the actor's behavior.

The basis for each of these components is a set of memories organizing our perceptions of the world around us and organizing our perceptions of the effects of our pursuing (or predicting the effects of someone else's pursuing) particular courses of action in the surrounding situation.

While all four components of someone's predicting someone else's behavior (or, to put that another way, our prediction of the results of his motivations) involve the situation, none of them involves it directly. The *situation* could alter markedly, in important or in trivial detail, without a change in perception, action, or prediction of action. And of course the *perception* of the situation may alter in some important detail for either the actor or predictor so that the prediction loses accuracy without any change having taken place in the external situation.

Without deviating from our central pursuit, which is to detail how the clinician perceives and deals with the patient's motivations, we can point out that the fourfold scheme for predicting the behavior of another person deals with the same kind of processes we have been dealing with in our considerations of all aspects of clinical decisions. We must deal with decisions based upon our sets of distributions of past events (memories) wherein the decisions are reached on the basis both of the memories of the outside world (which we are presently labeling situations) and memories of the importance to ourselves and to the actor of one kind of decision or another, each with its associated action.

We have gone onto the subject of motivation and action because we were inquiring into the question of how much a patient's perception of his own speech might be altered before he drops out of therapy. What we seemed to conclude in our tangential discussion is that human behavior is usually relatively simple and open to simple control. If behavior is open to easy prediction and simple control, then we should be careful in clinical interactions with patients. Particular care must be paid in early interaction lest we find that we, perhaps, alter the patient's perceptions of his own speech to his detriment before we have any reasonable understanding of his perceptions. Any clinician, in an interaction with a patient, carries an authority imputed to him by the patient that gives his remarks greater significance than the clinician-in-training typically realizes. Therefore, as has been mentioned, it can be expected that an offhand remark to the effect that his speech is "not too bad" might frequently result in the patient's permanent disappearance from the clinic before anyone has an opportunity to determine what the patient's perception of his own speech might be. Operationally, we can close consideration of the question as to how the patient's perception is influential in his pursuing therapy by recommending that when we want a patient to come for therapy, we need only positively reinforce his attendance behavior; when it is time to terminate, turn off the reinforcement for attendance and substitute reinforcers for termination.

Interestingly, while it is not adequately mentioned in the clinical literature, present evaluation techniques result in much the same conclusion. Contemporary techniques are not typically structured to explore patient's motivations, implying patients' behaviors are either generally open to simple control or unrelated to the therapy process.

We seem to have done an about-face. We began with an argument saying that one aspect of insight the clinician must obtain during an evaluation is the patient's payoff matrix, because it provides the medium for manipulating (or getting him to manipulate) his behavior. If speech behavior is open to relatively simple manipulation considering that the patient is already so motivated as to present himself for therapy, why explore his motivation?

There are two reasons to explore patient motivation. We already know that while behavior of another person can be predicted within some typical range, exact prediction requires a deeper knowledge of the actor. Second, we must engage in exact prediction because efficacious therapy is highly particularized to the patient (more precisely, to the patient-clinician interaction). Efficiency in therapy comes from competent use of idiosyncratic traits of the patient, and we must systematically explore his motivation during our evaluation to obtain the necessary knowledge for planning his therapy.

In general, given that the patient is open to relatively easy control (consciously or inadvertently) by the clinician or other persons in his environment, we reach the conclusion that the clinician should engage in quite conscious control of the patient's speech behavior by tying him to a schedule of various social reinforcers. The reinforcers should be designed, sequentially, to induce him to undertake an active role in therapy, to internalize the therapist's speech goals, and to terminate therapy with satisfaction in the therapeutic process and in his own speech when he achieves these goals.

We have said all we will say about evaluation of speech behavior. Perhaps some readers will wonder why we have talked about many aspects of the evaluation process but have not dealt at all with evaluation techniques. So now let us speak of these for a moment.

There is a wide variety of procedures and techniques used in evaluation. If we were to follow a particular clinician through his daily activities for an extended period, we should probably discover that he favors certain evaluative techniques, tests, and procedures, and uses them repeatedly. He may use others less often but on a recurring basis; some he uses not at all—indeed, he does not know them sufficiently well to use them with any confidence. But he does competent evaluations and we would have no fear about bringing a friend or relative to him for clinical diagnosis or therapy planning. If we followed a different clinician, we might discover he used some of the same techniques though his total set is quite different. But he also does competent evaluations and we would have equal confidence in him.

Any clinical evaluation is a more or less structured set of procedures to obtain an appropriate and sufficiently comprehensive observation set to allow the necessary decisions to be made with confidence. There are numerous ways of deriving the observation set, and no particular way can be considered best. What we must do is to find a way that is adequate and comfortable. So much of the teaching and development of the clinical skill of evaluation rests in the hands of our master supervising clinicians in university training programs that it would be presumptuous, even if possible, to try to put it into print.

We began by saying that our goal was to structure the clinical process. In the domain of a speech evaluation, we asserted that an evaluation requires securing five pieces of information, and we have spent some time discussing the reasons why we consider all five, and perhaps others, as necessary. To recapitulate, the five areas of knowledge are:

1. the clinician's perception of normal speech;
2. the clinician's perception of the patient's speech;
3. a prediction of appropriate and expected terminal behaviors;
4. components of the patient's motivation, including the patient's perception of normal speech and his perception of his own speech; and,
5. significant dyadic variables.

Audiological Evaluation

There are two attractive approaches we might use in dealing with evaluation in audiology. We can ask how our model might assist in structuring the things that *are* being done so as to increase their effectiveness. Alternatively, we can consider what *should* be the directions of audiologic evaluation, this last course of action presupposing some judgments about the "proper" role of audiology. Still other courses of action are open to us but consideration of just these two will be sufficient to delineate the available options provided by the model, so we shall do a bit of both.

Much of the argument in this chapter on evaluation has been couched in a style that seems to make it much more readily applicable to speech or language pathologies than to hearing impairments, and yet exactly the opposite should be the case. There is a sharper need for considering the structure of the evaluative process in hearing than in speech, if for no other reason than that we have come close here to losing our sense of direction.

The goal of an evaluation is to structure therapy—an obvious point that has already been commented upon. The goal is complex because much therapy *for* speech or hearing problems is not necessarily therapy *in* speech or hearing. The so-called cleft palate evaluation team has speech adequacy as a goal—one of several—and the evaluation by the speech examiner on the team may be of major importance in the final decision as to the therapeutic regime for the patient. But that therapeutic regime may involve no speech therapy at all. This seems to be true in audiology in particular.

PHILOSOPHICAL BASES OF PRESENT AUDIOLOGY PROCEDURES

There is a strong school of thought in contemporary audiology that finds two major roles for the audiologist. The first of these roles is to assist in the evaluative process to focus direction for medical or surgical therapy. The other role is that of engaging directly in one portion of the therapy process—hearing-aid fitting. The phrase *hearing-aid fitting* is used in preference to *hearing-aid evaluation* to reinforce the basic contention that we evaluate people and we do so in order to focus their therapy as meaningfully and economically as we can. This therapy may include "fitting" a patient with a hearing aid. But as therapists, we fit hearing aids to people; we have little interest in evaluating hearing aids.

This is not to suggest that hearing-aid research is meaningless. There may be much merit in attempting to discover physical characteristics of aids which will be found to relate to some audiologic measures on patients so that we can have reasonable general guidelines for increasing the efficiency of fittings. But at the time of this writing, no such data exist.

The interested reader should refer to Chapter 6, in which there is a discussion of the issue of hearing-aid fitting. The point to be made here is that current research and clinical practices in audiology are directed into two channels: evaluation for structuring nonaudiologic therapy, and evaluation for engaging in electro-acoustic therapy. You will note that both lines of activity in audiology are designed to depersonalize the patient. The more one considers the particular details of audiologic evaluation or hearing-aid fitting therapy, the more apparent this statement becomes. The evaluative process is less than adequate, if one listens to his audiologic colleagues, to the extent that it is contaminated by the conscious processes in the individual—by decision processes in the patient.

For example, there is significant interest in various procedures for objectifying audiometry so that the examiner can appraise the acuity of the "auditory system." The auditory system is somehow conceptualized as being independent of the rest of the nervous system in which it resides because the intention is to keep the patient from being able to fool the examiner. The examiner's purported goal is to obtain a measure of what the patient *can* hear whether the patient *does* hear it or not.

It sounds somewhat silly even to try to verbalize such a goal because taking it out of the technical terminology in which it typically is stated spotlights the incongruity, considered from the point of view of evaluation for therapy, of evaluating someone's *hearing* to which he does not or cannot admit. We shall return to this point, but first let us look at the other aspect of audiology—hearing-aid fitting.

Audiologic endeavors in hearing-aid fitting and use have, like audiologic evaluation, concentrated on depersonalization. To determine if he is a candidate, the patient is evaluated by use of monosyllabic words so that differences in listening strategy, intelligence, or educational level will be minimized in their influence on test results. If the examiner considers a patient may be influenced by instrument size, for example, many clinicians will structure the hearing aid fitting so that the patient does not see the instrument. Consciously or unconsciously, the point of view has been nourished in audiology that the less the results of any procedure are influenced by the idiosyncracies of the individual patient, the more scientific would be the discipline and the clinical examination.

There now seem to be two issues at cross-purpose—on the one hand, the audiologist assumes the responsibility for estimating the integrity of the auditory system, even for patients who may find it advantageous to exaggerate their social hearing difficulty; on the other hand, the audiologist realizes that there is little if any relation between any measures he might be able to obtain without the patient's cooperation (called "objective measures") and how well the patient may be said to hear in his typical activities of daily living. The clinician realizes that he must have reasonable cooperation to obtain any meaningful evaluation, when evaluation is considered a preliminary to therapy.

Our present concern is with the latter type of evaluation. The former type, which offers appraisal of the patient's acuity even in the absence of his cooperation, is of no present interest to us and will be dealt with in Chapter 6. The stress in this part of our presentation, as in all current speech evaluation procedures and in virtually every other clinical area, is the necessity to discover those aspects of behavior unique to the patient under evaluation. Not acuity, not discrimination for isolated monosyllabic words of high familiarity, not change in skin resistance mediated by involuntary changes in the autonomic nervous system, not changes in surface-measured electrical activity of the brain, but dimensions of behavior related to the therapeutic process.

UTILITY OF CURRENT PROCEDURES

All of this denotes a strongly negative reaction to many particular evaluative procedures in clinical audiology. Does this mean that we think all the evaluative procedures of current audiology are useless? Certainly not. It seems necessary to point up the peculiar direction in which audiology seems to have wandered, because we must become aware first that there is a problem. Until we are, we are likely to be lulled by our two decades of prolific output and technological development in audiology. We have made so much progress it is almost a foregone conclusion that what we have accomplished is both good and proper.

So let us go back to a restatement of the reason for any evaluation: to zero in on therapy, and reexamine the components of current audiologic appraisal.

We begin by considering lip-reading, or speech-reading ability. With virtually any present test of speech-reading ability available, we could find many persons showing highly similar results from testing and highly dissimilar social adequacy using their speech-reading abilities.

Why should this be so? We can think of speech-reading ability as being distributed in the population in a normal (chance) manner because it has a large number of independent components. Let us further assert that the ability can be considered as being open to evaluation on a single-dimension axis so that we should be able to build a reasonable test yielding a simple index of speech-reading ability. Accept the assertion for a moment so that we can use it as a springboard for a few other statements. Realize, however, that though the statements are highlighted by that assertion, the assertion is not necessary to them.

> A test of speech-reading is a model of speech-reading ability as the patient does, or potentially will, practice it, and because the test is a model it should be evaluated by a criterion of utility. However, *current tests of speech-reading ability do not relate in any simple way to day-by-day speech-reading ability.* That is, they have little if any utility.
>
> General audiologic evaluative procedures, as they are routinely conducted almost everywhere in this country, are equally useless for predicting speech-reading success.
>
> One cannot predict success in auditory training from either current tests of auditory training ability or routine (nonexceptional) tests used in audiologic assessment. They are useless.
>
> Exactly comparable statements can be made for therapeutic practices in speech conservation. Evaluation procedures predicting speech conservation success or directing therapy, if they exist at all, are useless.
>
> Frankly, in the overall picture, exactly the same statements apply to a very significant proportion of patients subjected to hearing-aid fitting procedures, done by either a hearing-aid dealer or an audiologist.

In sum, audiologic evaluative procedures seem to bear little relevance to any of the audiologic therapies. Does this mean that medical or surgical procedures have made audiologic therapy procedures superfluous? Hardly. For all of the dramatic advances of medicine over the past thirty years, there are more than twenty million persons handicapped in hearing who would be happy to testify to their social inadequacies.

Does it mean that there is no relevance to audiologic therapy? Again, the answer must be an emphatic No. What it does mean is that there is little relationship between formalized audiologic assessment and audiologic therapy, so that the individual clinician is more or less successful depending upon the additional observations he makes and the individual insight with which he interprets his observations. In other words, audiologic evaluation is a highly complex process and very little of the observational material necessary to these clinical decisions arises from the formalized results of audiologic assessments.

Appropriate Evaluation Goals

If it is true that, for directing the thrust of therapy, little of value arises from the typical complete audiologic assessment, one can legitimately ask what insights our model might provide toward clarifying this complex issue. Does our simple structure offer anything of value toward increasing the effectiveness of evaluation procedures in clinical audiology?

At an overview, the needs to be met by an audiologic assessment, seen from the point of view of the therapist interested in maximizing the communication performance of the patient, seem to be three: to evaluate the individual's present capacity for receiving communication; to evaluate the individual's potential for communication as it might differ from his present abilities because of therapies of one type or another; and to evaluate the individual's potential for communication as it might differ from his present abilities because of progression of the pathology or pathologies. To deal with the audiologic assessment in more detail it is necessary that we first delineate our goals for audiologic therapy.

Man uses his hearing for a wide variety of purposes that are more or less necessary to his survival and psychological well-being. Two of these are of primary importance: (1) the use of hearing as a warning system, and (2) the use of the auditory channel as an information receiver and processor. Both of these primary uses can be accomplished successfully by the person who hears in only one ear. But both are facilitated by having two-eared hearing. Binaural hearing results in man's having a sense of direction; the listener uses the differences in the sound coming to the two ears to orient himself to the direction (and distance) of the source. In circumstances of multiple sources, binaural abilities result in our separating the several sources and attending to one or to a selected few while giving little heed to the others. The process of focusing attention on a sound to the exclusion of other sources literally has the same effect as multiplying the sound pressure of the source by as much as fifteen times its actual value. In other words, our two ears give us the ability to localize sounds we choose to attend to—focusing on that sound by squelching other competitive sounds, we make a gain in loudness that we could get with only one ear by holding all the other sources at their original loudness and multiplying the sound pressure of the attended source by a factor of approximately fifteen. Obviously, then, therapy should be so dimensionalized as to come as close to restoring binaural hearing for the patient as we can get.

General goals for audiologic therapy are to maximize, within the limitations of the patient, his use of hearing as a nondirectional environmental monitoring system, and as an information receiver and processor. Both of these general goals count heavily upon the binaural system for their attainment, so establishment of normal binaural balance is a component of our general goal structure.[2]

Effective therapy must be structured to maximize the patient's use of his hearing as it might be, as well as his hearing as it is, so that a goal in evaluation is the ability to predict the possibility of a dynamic condition, and in that case, the rate and direction of change in acuity.

The sounds that alert us to danger and to desirable sound sources are too widely divergent in their characteristics in all three acoustic domains (frequency, amplitude, and time) for us to be able to describe other than their statistical characteristics. One can only specify minimum limits of resolution and range in any of the three domains necessary to normal performance. We tend, therefore, to forego consideration of these with the idea that if the individual can process speech signals, he can process alerting signals also.

Unfortunately, this last statement hardly clarifies the specification task. Speech also exists only statistically in that one cannot write a statement detailing the acoustic requirements for speech other than in a probabilistic sense. Certainly, one can write rules that would, on the average, indicate a particular utterance, but he cannot write the rules specifying the range of utterances that would be so identified. Of course, we have often made the point that what an individual identifies is, to a marked degree, determined by what he expects to identify and what he expects not to identify and the statement can be applied to speech as easily as to other complex signals. That is, his identifications are determined by his sets of distributions and his locations of his fences. This means that part of the structure of any speech message is in the listener before the speech ever gets there; we shall come back to this in the chapter on research implications.

Assuming that a goal of therapy is to maximize the patient's ability

[2] There is some recent work (D. W. Batteau, R. L. Plante, R. H. Spencer, W. E. Lyle, *Auditory Perception*. China Lake, Calif.: U. S. Naval Ordnance Test Station, Contract No. N123–(60530) 35401A, United Research Inc., Cambridge, 1964) suggesting that monaural processing may provide all the information necessary to equal binaural performance in source azimuth, signal separation, and the like, but this discussion will hold to the more accepted position that the binaural system, i.e., the second ear, is essential to successful performance in such decision tasks.

to process speech and assuming speech to be a statistical quantity, there seem to be two alternative routes to use in estimating a patient's present and potential ability to process speech. The first of these is the direct approach of using a sample of speech materials of such a magnitude and composition that one can draw meaningful conclusions about the patient's abilities to process the varieties of speech he will have to process in *his* day-to-day activities.

The alternative is to use some reductionist approach and appraisal technique: to assert that there are some few specific abilities necessary to processing speech; for example, temporal resolution of thirty milliseconds or better, or a dynamic range of amplitude (from barely detected to too painful) of greater than twenty decibels. The examiner can then appraise each of these abilities, weight each of the component results, and combine them to obtain a speech-intelligence estimate.

Either approach—testing speech hearing ability by using speech tests or testing that same ability by testing the few (?) specific abilities necessary to processing speech—highlights the importance of decision processes in the patient. The patient more willing to guess about a signal not clearly heard will be more often both right and wrong than another patient suffering equal lack of clarity but who is less willing to hazard any guess. Planning and executing successful therapy requires the knowledge that the patients have equal lack of clarity (or equal sensitivity) and the fact that the patients differ markedly in their relative willingness to guess and be wrong (the willingness to false alarm).

Because the presence of the patient in the evaluation procedure makes it likely that some loss of hearing for speech is present, the evaluator routinely must be prepared to appraise the patient's potential for rehabilitation and to seek, among the strategies of therapy that are available, those that appear to show most promise for optimizing his communication performance.

Finally, one must evaluate the patient's competence in processing signals coming from various locations, sequentially or simultaneously.

We have listed the following items for appraisal:

1. The patient's hearing for speech, monaurally in each ear.
   a) The examination may appraise primitive abilities underlying speech, or may appraise hearing for speech directly, or both
   b) The examination should include but separate acuity from decision

behavior in order to be able to estimate the effectiveness of the patient in utilizing the information he does receive
2. The direction and rapidity of expected physiological change in each ear
3. The advantage to the patient of binaural hearing—current status and predicted maximum
4. The patient's potential maximum performance following therapy
5. Determination of available therapeutic strategies and the options (including their respective payoff matrices) for patient and clinician

While there may be many other therapy requests from an individual patient for which some appraisal is necessary (for example, improving hearing of music, or making all sounds softer), the typical evaluation need involve itself with only the above components as its core.

We indicated earlier that it would be appropriate to appraise listener capacities for warning signals as well as for speech signals. For economy of time, we can probably use some indices taken during testing of the patient's hearing of speech to assist us in appraising his hearing capacities for various types of environmental signals.

INADEQUACIES IN CURRENT AUDIOLOGICAL ASSESSMENTS

Let us now take a few pages to spell out more of the implications of our audiologic evaluation model, primarily by contrast with current assessment procedures. As presently undertaken, a typical evaluation involves a short history oriented toward symptomatology, identification data, and history of progression of the loss. Symptomatology and progression of loss both relate to item 2 of our appraisal schedule: the direction and rapidity of expected physiological change. We should, however, note that symptomatology and progression of loss have audiological as well as medical therapy components, even though too frequently in current practice the questionnaire contains much information of direct use to the otologist but of little value to the audiologic therapist.

The second part of the typical assessment is a pure-tone audiogram. Many audiologic clinics undertake to estimate monaural acuity for frequencies in the range 250 Hz (or 125 Hz) through 4000 Hz (or even 8000 or 10,000 Hz) at half-octave locations, monaurally for each ear by air conduction and by bone conduction. Some clinics will undertake part or all of the same task as an addition to or substitute for discrete frequency audiometry, by use of a continuous frequency Békésy tracing for continuous and/or pulsed presentation of tones. When a cooperative patient who has some hearing loss is given good instructions, the clinician derives re-peatable pure-tone "thresholds" in about an hour. The subject of tonal audiometry is examined in detail in Chapter 6. Let us examine it now in a cursory fashion to evaluate its contribution to planning therapy. An audiogram is administered by delivering signals of varying durations with intermixed varying delays. When a signal is delivered, the examiner credits the patient with hearing it if the patient so indicates. But the examiner asserts the patient heard nothing if the examiner delivered a signal and the patient made no response. The clinician, generally speak-ing, ignores responses of the patient when no signal is delivered (false alarms) though repeated false alarms may cause him to think the patient has a hallucinatory problem.

If we consider a test that both presents and withholds signals while giving the patient a choice of response, then we have four possibilities. The patient can say "signal" when there was or was not a signal, and he can say "no signal" when there was or was not a signal. For the patient to be able to respond "no signal" he must have some idea of the interval during which a signal can appear if it is to appear at all.

In the audiogram test, the patient can say "signal" and that is all. The audiologist ignores false alarms and, because the patient is never given an observation interval, the patient can say "no signal" repeatedly or not at all. So what an audiogram represents is the willingness of any patient to guess about the presence of a signal. An audiogram, therefore, may tell us a great deal that is therapeutically useful about guessing be-havior (decision behavior) of a patient or it may tell us nothing. Un-fortunately, we have never done the kinds of studies on audiometry with clinical patients to allow us to know what aspects of decision information the examination may contain. But an audiogram must be suspect as a measure of the sensitivity of a patient about whom we are trying to get insights for planning therapy. It may or may not be a reasonable estimate of some kind of sensitivity of the auditory system, but it seems to give us little insight for planning audiologic therapy for the patient.

Certainly, the audiologist often serves as a supplier of information to a physician who will add additional information to make a decision con-cerning medical or surgical treatment. And for these decision makers the audiogram appears to have high utility. But our concern is our own role in therapy, and an evaluative regime is judged by us from its utility for audiologic therapy. Given this goal, the audiogram gives us little return for so great an investment in time.

Subsequent to obtaining an audiogram from a patient, we typically come to some measure of the patient's performance using speech signals. In the overwhelming majority of audiologic assessments this measure is derived by delivering a monosyllabic word signal to the listener from a tape- or phonograph-stored set and allowing him to select a response from his own internal lexicon. We score the word as correct if it agrees with the word printed on the piece of paper in front of the tester.

The point is that we are trying to obtain several things, and notable among them is an estimate of present and future binaural processing of speech in the daily environment of the patient. What contribution an index of monosyllabic word recognition may make toward that estimate can be answered only empirically. The nature of current clinical tasks intermixes the patient's ability to get cues from a speech signal delivered through his impaired system with his strategies—in using those cues to decide upon his response, once he gets them. Because we do not know what cues he does and does not get, because we do not know the exact set of responses from among which he chooses the response he delivers, and because we do not know what kinds of rules make up his decision strategy, we cannot derive a great deal of information about his ability to process speech in his typical environment, and this last is precisely the rationale for giving the test in the first place.

We have implied that many factors influence any person's performance on a word test. These factors have been studied most insightfully by many persons, most notably Goldiamond,[3] and the interested reader will find this and additional references in the bibliography. (In addition, see "Research on Audiologic Evaluation, Chapter 6).

All other testing procedures in the armamentarium of the audiologist seem to represent sophisticated procedures either to test the patient who is suspected of feigning some portion of his loss or to enhance the knowledge underlying a medical or surgical decision. It seems not unreasonable to conclude that the development of audiology in recent years has been primarily and almost completely from an acute-disease orientation rather than a more appropriate chronic-disease orientation. The climate in which the audiologist functions can be characterized by a philosophy of immediate treatment, expressed sometimes through surgery, sometimes through hearing-aid fitting with little follow-up of associated therapy. Long-term hearing rehabilitation languishes for lack of interest, lack of research, and lack of persons being adequately trained.

[3] I. Goldiamond, "Perception," in A. Bachrach, ed. *The Experimental Foundations of Clinical Psychology* (New York: Basic Books, 1963).

Components of an Audiological Assessment

What should be the components of an audiological assessment of specific interest to the hearing therapist? Let us, in considering the question, completely bypass those aspects of an assessment needed for evaluation of a pathology or its progression. Such interests are well represented in our everyday clinical activities so we will do them no injustice in ignoring them temporarily.

First of all, the individual patient's capacities, the training strategies, and so forth—all those things that most radically influence the course of therapy—must somehow get thrust into the evaluation matrix. While evaluation of the patient's capacities is a desirable goal, it will be a confusing and perhaps overwhelming task if it does not reflect the relative importance of such characteristics to the communication functioning of the patient. Therefore it must be accompanied by a systematic appraisal of such things as the demands imposed by various environments, sizes of groups, and background noise levels. This seems to coalesce to a new attempt to develop a measure of social adequacy for hearing modeled on the philosophic approaches underlying the text *Hearing and Deafness,* particularly Ramsdell's chapter,[4] and the original work on the Social Adequacy Index by Davis.[5] This is not to suggest that it might be possible to derive a single number estimate of a patient's social adequacy, for indeed I think this is unlikely, but we must structure our thinking about the demands made by various communication interactions so that we can focus on optimizing the patient's abilities to meet these demands.

Whether we should use procedures that sample various speech types or procedures that sample reductionist measures of performance purported to underlie speech (such as dynamic range of loudness) was a question we raised earlier. It does not seem necessary to make a strong commitment to either course of action to the exclusion of the other, but it should be noted that the former position should allow a simultaneous appraisal of the listening strategies that the patient tends to employ in the situations under test. By the same token, one might employ a procedure that builds artificial speech context in order to appraise listener

---

[4] H. Davis and S. R. Silverman, *Hearing and Deafness,* Third ed. (New York: Holt, 1970), see esp. D. A. Ramsdell, "The Psychology of the Hard-of-Hearing and the Deafened Adult," in Davis and Silverman, *Hearing and Deafness.*
[5] H. Davis, "The Articulation Area and the Social Adequacy Index for Hearing," *The Laryngoscope,* 58 (1948), 761–778.

strategies (as well as to train listeners in optimal strategies), and work of this nature has recently been thoughtfully begun by Speaks.[6]

The testing protocols that must be developed for the above purposes will include testing under various binaural listening conditions, probably both at what would be a typical speech-loudness level for that circumstance (that is, some specified Hearing Level) and at what would be an appropriate level for that person (some specified Sensation Level or definition of Comfort Level). It will be necessary that we pursue studies on several aspects of the dimensions being suggested, in particular studies dealing with the implications of different levels of hearing in the two ears (for a beginning attack on this problem, see Heffler and Schultz [7]).

Finally, we must find ways to appraise the additional information contributed to the perceiver when he can utilize nonauditory inputs as a supplement to his hearing.

Many of these goals for a comprehensive hearing evaluation, of use in focusing hearing therapy, are pursued in more detail in later sections, particularly in Chapter 6.

Our orientation throughout this presentation assumes that a received message is understood partially on the basis of the expectations of the person doing the receiving. Only with the exercise of great caution can we study normals to help us understand pathologicals if persons with impaired hearing are systematically different in their expectations than persons with normal hearing. Routine attempts to predict results from pathologicals on the basis of extrapolation from results on normals will probably markedly oversimplify the problem and lead to misdirected effort and inefficient research.[8]

[6] C. E. Speaks, "Synthetic-Sentence Identification and the Receiver Operating Characteristics," *Journal of Speech and Hearing Research,* 10 (1967), 110–119.

[7] A. J. Heffler and M. C. Schultz, "Some Implications of Binaural Signal Selection for Hearing-Aid Evaluation," *Journal of Speech and Hearing Research,* 7 (1964), 279–289.

[8] M. C. Schultz and M. S. Berman, "Speech Recognition Behavior in normals and Otopathological Persons," *Journal of Speech and Hearing Research,* in press.

FOUR

Clinical Therapy Procesess

Therapy Concepts

We have laid down the major ground rule for therapy in the preceding chapter, while defining the components of evaluation: a therapy procedure implies primary information flow from the therapist to the patient. We have even gone farther and presented some of the kinds of knowledge that must be transmitted in this interpersonal communication process we call therapy. The therapist must give the patient (that is, somehow cause the patient to accept and internalize) appropriate speech goals.

We can now characterize appropriate speech goals as coming from a dual perception on the part of the clinician. One major determiner of appropriate (or adequate, or acceptable) speech is society's criterion for acceptable speech, so that the clinician must monitor this facet in determining his criterion. It would be totally inappropriate for a therapist from one dialect region to be so chauvinistic as to apply his societal patterns of articulation to patients in another dialect region, but this should not prevent the therapist from having such a criterion or from using it when appropriate. The second force in selecting adequate speech goals for a patient is a consideration of the patient's competence for achieving culturally acceptable speech. An individual who does not have the potential for achieving an acceptable level of nasality in his vocal quality must come to realize and accept his own nasality as minimized by therapy even though he may realize that this performance is highly atypical.

Two cautions are appropriate appendages to this last paragraph. First, the clinician must come to therapy with an excellent perception of the normal distribution on various speech qualities, both as regards the mean and the variance. This has significant implications for training and is covered in that section. Secondly, the decision that a patient has a particular potential level of competence for some speech or hearing characteristic is a decision by the therapist, and it is no more than a prediction.

There will be two kinds of labeling errors in the repeated performances of the clinician making such predictions. Some patients will have goals of adequate speech set for them that they cannot achieve; others will be encouraged to accept their own speech when it is less adequate than they or society would like, and less than they can reasonably achieve. The therapist must be aware that such errors of judgment are unavoidable, but he should continually strive to minimize them. Also, he should probably be more willing to make an error of omission (saying the patient can do no better when he can) than an error of commission (saying that patient can do better when he cannot).

However, the clinician must be careful that he does not establish goals for the patient that are less than culturally satisfactory and less than reasonable for the patient. While it is better to err in this direction than the others, errors should be minimized. The therapist must be a source of inspiration for the patient so that the patient strives to please him. In later stages of therapy, the patient should have internalized the evaluative criteria of the therapist and should be getting enough appropriate feedback from his daily environment that the therapist's influence decreases in importance for acquisition and maintenance of communication skills. But early in therapy, the therapist represents the primary source of critical judgment of progress and of the closing gap between current status and final speech or hearing goals. The therapist always has the responsibility of shifting the critical judgment from himself to society in general or, in selected situations wherein the patient cannot expect to achieve "acceptable" speech standards, to the patient. If the therapist does not meet this responsibility, the patient cannot have a firm foundation for terminating therapy.

All the remaining components of therapy are reasonably derived from our model but we shall display them for purposes of further discussion.

With respect to appropriate speech goals, the therapist must supply an appropriate decision axis; he must educate the patient in those qualities of his (the patient's) speech or hearing to which he must attend if he is to accomplish the necessary discriminations. Applying an appropriate decision axis, typically, is not especially difficult although like many other persons who come late to a field without closely questioning all of its bases, we tend to fall heir to a kind of brainwashing from time to time. Consider, for a moment, the case of articulation therapy. The patient considers himself more or less intelligible (clear, understandable) though we characterize him as having a greater or lesser articulation problem. To my knowledge, the only person to have addressed himself to consideration of the relationship between these two is Guttman [1], following a line of work he began some years ago with Fairbanks [2]. But it certainly is necessary that someone address himself to: (1) the relationship between severity of misarticulation and intelligibility, or (2) the relationship between the attractiveness of a misarticulation (its ability to call attention to itself) and the intelligibility of the message from which it distracts or (3) the relationship between the difficulty of a misarticulation (its resistance to therapy) and its influence on intelligibility. Notice that two of these three possible issues cited for exploration may be of vital interest to us but they hold little interest for a patient. He does not care if we rate a /dʒ/ substitution and a /t/ substitution each as being a 3 or a 6. He may care that he cannot articulate either sound but one of them has a high frequency of occurrence in English, so that he has trouble with it all the time. The other sound occurs much less frequently and this articulation difficulty probably concerns him little, if at all.

There is no intention to assert that articulation therapy is inappropriate, for it may be precisely what is necessary. But there may be many children, for example, in articulation therapy who have significantly less communication difficulty than other children who are not in therapy but who have hoarse voices and are much less intelligible in a noisy classroom. Looked at in a slightly different way, there may be children in therapy for a series of articulation errors, but the phoneme undergoing change was chosen to give the child early success, even though it alters his intelligibility virtually not at all. Meanwhile, another phoneme awaits therapy because it is less tractable but, at the same time, the child would be easier to understand were this sound altered first. In this latter case, we might say the therapist is confusing success in therapy with success in communication. And we might even go so far as to assert that transfer would be no problem were the therapist to work on the latter phoneme first because of societal reward for better intelligibility, whereas

[1] N. Guttman, "Measurement of Articulatory Merit," *Journal of Speech and Hearing Research,* 9 (1966), 323–339, and "A Nomogram for the Articulatory Product," *Journal of Speech and Hearing Research,* 10 (1967), 311–312.
[2] G. Fairbanks, *Experimental Phonetics: Selected Articles* (Urbana: University of Illinois Press, 1966).

the therapy on the former phoneme has no genuine payoff outside of the therapy session and may never be generalized.

Much of this section, on the general definition of therapy, is expressed in terms of gross distributions on, for example, speech articulations. However, defining a decision axis requires consideration of particulars. In production of the phoneme /p/ for example, we are aware that a microscopic evaluation shows normal production of this phoneme in various contexts to be more than a single distribution. As an instance, the /p/ is articulated with aspiration in the prevocalic position (before a vowel in the same syllable) but without aspiration in the post-vocalic position. This general rule is adequate unless the /p/ is clustered, as in 'spit' because in this position also there is no aspiration. Therefore, it is not only necessary that we define the gross distribution that encompasses the phoneme /p/, but we must also give our patient some appreciation of its microscopic anatomy of articulation, or we will discover a significant problem in getting him to "transfer" what he has learned in therapy— through isolated productions—to its use in the contextual speech of the everyday real world circumstance.

For persons who have articulation problems but not difficulties in auditory discrimination, it is also necessary that the therapist train the patient in bringing his sets of production distributions and his sets of reception distributions into congruence. The patient must hear his own speech as others hear him and as he hears the speech of others. This is probably most economically accomplished in the feedback about the patient's productions if the therapist responds in terms of an appropriate distribution; for example: "That was acceptable though barely within normal range"; "That was better than necessary"; and so forth. This should assist the patient in determining the average and the range for an appropriate (therapist-defined) normal distribution.

The state of the patient will be altered by having the therapist provide a model (ideal) for the patient. The specifics of providing such a model are open to discussion and future research (Does one provide only a mean target value? Does one accept any production, no matter how poor, that is better than the previous production? Does one "shape" productions?) but as a central concept, there must be feedback from a reliable and valid judge of output—a therapist.

Associated with the definition of a normal distribution, as delineated by the therapist for the patient, should be an accompanying definition of the limits of the criterion for the normal distribution, so that the patient achieves a sharp delineation of this fence. There seems to be a natural tendency in most of us to shy away from a fence, to allow some margin of safety, so that providing a clearly delineated fence should assist the patient in moving toward adequate production.

Establishing a reasonable range for the normal distribution and a sharp delineation of the fence requires providing a large number of experiences for the patient so that a criterion of effective therapy should be magnitude of output of the speech under therapy. As professionals, we must concentrate on those techniques that maximize performance by the patient and this must be a goal and a criterion for effective therapy.

It probably is unnecessary to repeat that a high output means a high rate of error. It does not necessarily mean a high proportion of error, but the greater the output the greater the absolute number of errors. We must therefore be prepared for errors both as clinicians and as patients. This implies that the clinician must reward good performance without penalizing poor performance. Do not penalize it but do not reward it. We know that if someone can increase his winnings by guessing in a game, he will do so. But if guessing and being wrong costs him too much, he will reduce his guessing (shift his criterion). If he reduces his guessing, he will keep his hit proportion high and reduce the overall number of hits because he will respond only when he can be reasonably sure he is correct. But in our case, this is not what the clinician desires. What we want is for him to produce a very high output. We should therefore reinforce only those productions meeting our criteria, and the faster he produces, the faster he can internalize our criterion.

TWO PRINCIPLES GUIDING THERAPY

Before dimensionalizing therapy by use of the model, let us interject two characteristics important to the therapy process but not restricted to it. First, *we do not unlearn anything!* We may forget a behavior; more likely we may superimpose another behavioral repertoire over the first so that we no longer engage in the earlier behavior, but we do not unlearn it. If an individual is engaging in behavior we consider not appropriate to his speech or his clinical behavior, saying "stop" is not an appropriate instruction. One must teach the patient a substitution behavior, one must give reinforcement encouraging (rewarding) the new behavior, and one must not reinforce the old behavior. And, because the therapist does not control the milieu of the patient for more than a very few minutes per week and because too many persons in the surroundings of the patient will unwittingly reinforce the older undesired behavior, the therapist must get an exceptionally high number of new behavior responses with high reinforcement into the output of the patient when he is in therapy. The new behavior must displace the old behavior because the old behavior is always there to be used if the environment will reinforce it.

The other behavioral principle is that we are not consistent in our reactions, beliefs and the like. This is not meant in the obvious sense that we show lack of consistency in performance, but rather that we hold mutually incompatible views at one and the same time. Shall we say that, as human beings, we seem not to be wholly rational at times? We know that patients sometimes do things that are antagonistic to their own best interests, and we know that we sometimes do things in therapy that are not to the patient's interests—things that are not in the direction of improvement in therapy. In order to protect ourselves in the light of these inconsistent actions we fall into a kind of imperception about our own behavior and that of persons around us. In this way we shield ourselves from facing those personal inconsistencies. But if we are going to have to motivate our patients to produce a high speech output and if we are going to have to reward those productions that meet our criteria and withhold reinforcement from those productions that do not meet our criteria, then we are going to have to define what we will accept as appropriate productions and maintain high vigilance with respect to their occurrence. Previously, we indicated that impressing new habits as replacements for old ones requires a high production out put from the patient. High vigilance, also, is most easily maintained with high output so that, again, the importance of high performance by the patient must be stressed.

In addition, sometimes the therapist must deal with a patient who is not motivated—one who finds himself in the situation because of conditions beyond his control. For such persons, the therapist must provide such control of the therapy situation as to motivate his patient toward accomplishment of his (the patient's) role in therapy. To do so requires that the patient provide some indication of that state and the more output he renders, the better the therapist's estimation of it and the faster it can be altered. This means that any technique that increases the output by a certain amount, other things being equal, is better than any technique increasing output by less than that particular amount.

The techniques for accomplishing this task may be considered an extension of our model but are not explained by the model. These techniques derive from behavioral engineering—behavioral control through stimulus control and contingency management—and though such considerations are not at deviance with our model, it is not appropriate that we discuss them in the present context. (The interested reader is referred to Holland and Skinner,[3] Homme,[4] and Premack.[5] For applications to our field, see the recent work of Garrett [6] and his group at New Mexico State University.)

Therapy has one additional goal, which has already been discussed but should be restated. This is to prepare the patient to terminate therapy. Therapy must seek its own cessation.

Application of the Model to Therapy

The implications of the model may be particularized for therapy by dealing separately with therapy operations involving individual components of the model. We will sequentially consider the decision axis, the distribution parameters of mean and variance, and the location of criteria. Finally, we will deal with some general considerations displaying the utility of modeling to determine what options are available to the therapist dealing with various communication problems.

CHANGING THE DECISION AXIS

Therapy operates, in the main, by increasing distinctiveness. Within the conceptual scheme of our model, this can be achieved in a variety of ways. One can increase the knowledge base on the decision axis by increasing the factors influencing the decision variable. That is to say, the patient can be taught to be perceptive of characteristics previously not noted with the idea that the distributions on the new decision axis will

[3] J. G. Holland and B. F. Skinner, *Analysis of Behavior: Programmed Instruction* (New York: McGraw-Hill, 1961).

[4] L. E. Homme, "Contiguity Theory and Contingency Management," *The Psychological Record*, 16 (1966), 233–241.

[5] D. Premack, "Reinforcement Theory," in D. Levine, ed., *Nebraska Symposium on Motivation* (Lincoln: University of Nebraska Press, 1965).

[6] E. R. Garrett, *Speech and Language Therapy Under an Automated Stimulus Control System*. Final Report, Project No. 3192, Contract No. OE–6–10–198, New Mexico State University, January 1968.

be more discrete than on the present axis. This would be the goal of new screening techniques for first graders, or the addition of a biopsy in the laryngological clinic. In such examples, one is obviously bringing more knowledge into consideration with the goal of sharpening the distinction between normal and pathological.

One is doing the same thing in recommending use of a *synthetic* approach rather than an *analytic* approach in speech-reading (lip-reading). A synthetic approach gives the speech reader a rationale for delaying his decisions about the incoming signals so that he maximizes the information base for his decisions. One way to conceptualize this example is to consider that a synthetic approach, by concentrating upon topic of conversation as a first decision, reduces the set of possible messages from one involving conversation about anything in the world of the talker (a very large, even potentially infinite, set) to some relatively small set of messages appropriate to that talker on that topic.[7] The central point for our present consideration is that there are varying ways in therapy of altering the decision axis to increase the distinctiveness of the perceived distributions, and differing occasions when it is proper to do so.

REDUCING THE VARIANCE

A second way of increasing distinctiveness is to decrease the variance in one or both distributions, thereby diminishing the magnitude of overlap. When should it be appropriate to consider this strategy? Exactly when one cannot deal with either the decision axis, per se, or alter the location of either distribution. This situation occurs when some pathology limits the spectrum of factors influencing the decision variable that is available to the patient.

One such striking example is seen in the following typical occurrence: those who have hearing impairments most often do not have auditory control mechanisms for speech that function adequately. This results in what might be viewed as an increase in the number of occurrences of speech productions that differ significantly from the ideal or target production and can be represented as a gradual elevation, over some long period of the loss, of one or both ends of the distribution representing

---

[7] Considered from the point of view of information theory also, synthetic rather than analytic speech-reading approaches have much to recommend them. This latter point of view is given explicit exposition in Chapter 6, page 128, covering implications of the model for research.

the sound complex. A very specific example might be the progressively greater intrusion of voicing into a typically unvoiced consonant, accompanied by a gradually increasing duration of the sound. In Figure 18, these distortions would tend to destroy the /f/–/v/ distinction. Note that

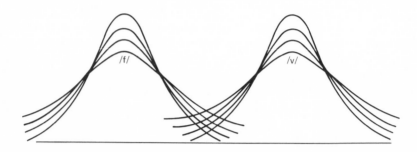

FIGURE 18. *Increase in variance in distributions of productions of two phonemes occurring over time because of loss af auditory feedback for control.*

the /v/ undergoes the same types of changes that may dissolve the distinction between it and some other sound, but would not assist in the /f/–/v/ distinction.

It would seem good therapy to try to give the patient much sharper lines of distinction by reducing the variability he allows in control of his own production of neighboring phonemes. While he may have significant difficulty in arriving at these more sharply separated distributions, as he will have to minimize some of the influences of phoneme environment that tend to increase variance in the speech-production distributions of normals, when he does achieve the variance reduction his cutoff will be in a location on the axis where neither /f/ nor /v/ is now produced. Except for rare productions, he and his listener will both be much more secure about phonemic distinctiveness as he generates them in the future.

As Figure 19 illustrates, it is much easier to maintain a distinction in 19B than in 19A, for in the situation depicted in A, high hit rates (calling a /v/ a /v/) necessarily are accompanied by some reasonable level of false alarms (calling an /f/ a /v/), so the distinction is already cloudy. Note that the therapy is not designed to do anything but reduce the variability of the patient's production distributions, even though this is no simple task. In so doing, however, the therapist significantly reduces the false alarm rate for any given hit rate, and increases the distinctiveness with respect to the patient's own ability to monitor his output and with respect to the listener's ability to understand the spoken message.

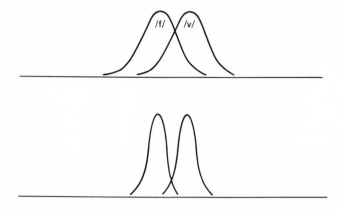

FIGURE 19. *Increase of discriminability of productions of two phonemes because of more stringent control of allowable variance.*

RELOCATING CRITERIA

Still a third procedure for increasing distributional distinctiveness therapeutically is to alter the mean location of one or both distributions. While this may be the procedure that seems most obvious when one is considering only the structure of the model, it is probably the least frequently occurring. Our early example of the young female stutterer brought in for evaluation represents such a strategy, as the problem arises probably from a misperception on the part of the parents as to the distributional aspects of nonfluencies. Their perception of pathological dysfluency as a distribution probably has a mean value much closer to the mean of the normal dysfluency distribution than was appropriate. Where the parent or patient is evaluating his distributions in most other conditions of interest in speech and hearing, such misperceptions tend not be so dramatic.

RELOCATING CRITERIA

In therapy one can determine that he need alter neither the decision axis nor either the means or variances of the distributions appearing on such axes, but that the patient must have his criterion relocated. Therefore, first let us reflect for a moment on what constitutes an adequate criterion.

Adequate criterion cutoffs—that is, adequate for use in production or reception in general societal communication—should be located in a way yielding minimal misunderstanding in the face of the large variability encountered in the speech of a wide variety of persons and situations. In normal learning, the listener is subjected to great variability and establishes such cuts with some reasonable knowledge of the distinctiveness of the distributions under consideration.

Our previous discussion of the microscopic anatomy of such a distribution as $/p/$ set the stage for our dealing with the location of an adequate criterion cutoff in therapy. An appropriate location of a cutoff for the nonclustered prevocalic $/p/$ has aspiration as part of the criterion variable, and the presence of some magnitude of aspiration weights the $/p/$ production so that it falls on the appropriate side of the fence. The use of a nonaspirated $/p/$ would result in a magnitude of the decision variable such that the production would fall to the other side of the fence, perhaps raising a question in the listener whether the talker has an "accent," or the phoneme was a $/b/$.

Different contexts result in systematic differences in microarticulation. Altering a phoneme (or some other unit of speech) considered defective must involve having the patient achieve satisfactory articulation in a variety of contexts, and we must appreciate that each context may differ in all allowable production variance. Within the framework of the therapy situation, however, the learner (the patient) is taught to produce the appropriate signal in a context exerting minimal influence toward increasing production variance. Many times, early therapy trials stress production in isolation. The model suggests one caution to be observed in this type of therapeutic strategy: the patient may be led to choose a fence that will be quite adequate for distinguishing these minimal context productions from his previous aberrant speech, but the fence may prove too stringent for contextual speech, which is influenced so much more by environment. If the patient is presented with the conflicts arising from acceptance of an unrealistic cut, therapy may prove to have been ineffective because the patient cannot maintain successful performance in contextual situations outside the therapy room.

A means of avoiding such a problem in transfer of training is to insure that the patient has wide experience in therapy with the variance in "normal" productions of the unit under therapeutic attack. It may seem inefficient, for example, to make the patient with a nasal voice try to achieve normal quality in utterances that have varying degrees of nasal assimilation. Indeed, the recognized clinical strategy seems to be to start him with sentences free of nasal assimilation altogether and only very slowly introduce nasal environments. Conceptually, it might be argued that in such an approach the patient is allowed to generate a tentative criterion as to his appropriate non-nasal quality, but with each additional therapeutic exposure to increasing amounts of unavoidable (that is, appropriate) nasal assimilation from context, he must shift his criterion fence back toward "nasality." How he arrives at some appropriate auditory memory of what should be the "normal" voice in the face of a constantly shifting criterion is difficult to understand. Perhaps a more effective strategy would be to establish a realistic fence for the patient by using varying contexts with more or less nasal assimilation from the begining of therapy. It may be true that the patient will have more trouble appreciating and achieving the finer discrimination, but the technique will have the major advantage of offering a criterion that is consistent as well as realistic.

It may have occurred to the reader that the criterion problem as much involves the typical therapist as the typical patient. We can illustrate this last point in a very simple manner. We have already mentioned several times that the appropriate description of a phoneme is a distribution, and some distributions on phonemes will overlap the distributions of their neighbors, as expressed by our predilection to misidentify them mutually. In Figure 20 we consider a pair of distributions

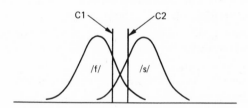

FIGURE 20. *Two criterial fences for accepting different phoneme productions during therapy.*

representing /f/ and /s/ and two different cutoffs, C1 and C2, for the placements of phones in these phonemes.

We may picture a clinician engaging in a process of speech stimulation with a young child. At some time during the set of therapy sessions in which the child will participate, he will be asked to produce a word or nonsense syllable containing an /f/ sound. The therapist will reward the child for any attempt to the left of C2. This allows the child much leeway in production attempts, maintains some reasonable criterion for /f/ phoneme productions with respect to the various environments and speakers that will cause phonetic variability in the sound produced in context, and still provides a criterion the clinician can use in deciding whether or not to reward the production attempt. All of these goals are appropriate. The reason that the therapy regime is less than adequate is that the clinician will tend to perform a comparable task in stimulating production of the /s/ phoneme, now using C1 as a cutoff.

The therapist does not realize the problem because he engages in each procedure individually, but the child must store and use two criteria that conflict with one another. Inevitably, the child will resolve the problem by realizing that both criteria are appropriate and that the area between C1 and C2 is sometimes heard as /f/ and sometimes as /s/, depending upon the environment. Until this realization strikes the child, he may be confused, and rightfully so, about the inconsistency of the therapist.

Perhaps a safer approach comes from pointing out that there is an inconsistency in labeling (this can be done by practice rather than by verbalization) that avoids needless confusion in the child. Either way, the model highlights the basic problem and its inevitability. Before leaving this example, it might be fruitful again to raise the question as to whether this labeling inconsistency may not be a large component in the transfer problem. The child may not use a sound learned as an isolated sound during therapy in his spontaneous conversation because the influences of phonetic environment would cause him to violate a clinically established and reinforced fence. The clinical criterion cutoff he has learned proves not good enough for the various contextual productions that involve greater variance. He cannot use his new single criterion so he chooses to revert to the older, even though unacceptable, pattern because both patterns give unacceptable productions. Caught between an older failing pattern and a newer failing pattern, he reverts to the older whose price he already knows.

ALTERNATE THERAPY STRATEGIES

What occurs in much of speech and hearing therapy is that one gives the patient more knowledge, more practice in hearing distinctions, and more practice in using physiological feedback. The patient learns to separate distributions and diminish errors, both misses and false alarms, without any need to alter his criteria. It seems reasonable to say that separation of distributions is the desirable aim and one that most therapists pursue without concerning themselves with any abstract model of therapy.

However, it is precisely in the case where the technique of separating distributions *cannot* be employed that the model becomes efficient, because it lights alternatives that are still open to the therapist.

When can the distinction between normal and pathological—between one speech sound and another—not be increased, and what are the alternatives open to the patient at that time?

The distributions cannot be altered when some limitation prevents the gaining of any further discrimination as, for example, in dysarthric articulation or speech discrimination with hearing loss. In these situations, there simply is not sufficient information that the patient can use to achieve the degree of separation obtained by the person with a nonorganic problem. It seems evident that the clinician should first maximize the cues that the patient can use effectively to reach as great a separation as he can achieve. It is also evident that this maximum discrimination will still yield some significant overlap with concomitant proportions of misses and false alarms.

When the therapist has accomplished a maximal sharpening of the discrimination of the patient, he should than attempt to maximize the hit rates for the degree of discrimination available to the patient. For a dysarthric patient, this means making him aware of the errors that must occur, because to maximize hit rates inevitably maximizes the false alarm rates. This strategy allows the patient to gain a healthy attitude toward his errors and makes him aware of the misinterpretations to which his speech may be open. He can then learn to take steps to minimize such confusions by repeating, paraphrasing, and the like. Therapy, in this situation, should include searching out the inevitable errors, estimating for the patient the percentage of time they will occur on the average, and their relative importance. How can the therapist assist the patient in searching out the errors of importance and dealing with them? One can estimate the percentage *occurrence* of an error by having the patient deliver a large sample of speech and simply counting the percentage of time that X is called Y, for every X and Y. The *importance* of the error on the average is probably related to the frequency of occurrence in general conversation of the sound on which the error is made. That is to say, a somehow misproduced /d3/ even half the time for this talker is of no consequence because of the low overall frequency of /d3/. But if the speaker misarticulates a /d/, which occurs about one in every twenty-five sounds, then his listener is exposed to potential misunderstanding four percent of the time.

Exactly the complement of this situation occurs with the hearing-handicapped person. To illustrate the problem and a strategy for solution, let us restrict our consideration to errors at a phoneme level, though there is no need to restrict ourselves to any particular size of unit, as the technique itself can be generalized.

The person whose hearing is handicapped can be thought of as having: no difficulty with many phonemes, difficulty in some contexts with some phonemes, and routine difficulty with nearly every occurrence of other phonemes. The first task in therapy is to maximize his discrimination for all phonemes, a task typically accomplished economically through the use of a standard learning paradigm: the patient receives a signal, responds to it, the response is evaluated and he is given feedback on the evaluation, and he is rewarded for correct performance. In our example, taken at the phoneme level, the therapist (or a surrogate) could deliver words to the patient, who repeats each. If the response is correct (matches the signal delivered, phoneme by phoneme), the word is struck from the list, the patient is told he was correct (which should serve as its own reward for adults), and the next word is delivered. If the word is incorrect, the patient is told he was incorrect and the word is repeated. If missed again, he is told again that it was incorrect and the word is re-repeated. If missed a third time, he is told what the word was by any means necessary to insure that he knows what it was, it is delivered a final time so that he can respond correctly, and the therapist moves to the next word.

If the therapist uses a list of, let us say, 500 words of common occurrence, he could go through the list in repeated therapy sessions, going back over any word not crossed out. A word is crossed out only if it was heard correctly on the first presentation of that use of the list. Successive uses are constrained to words incorrectly perceived in previous presentations so that gradually the therapist moves to phonemes frequently misperceived.

For many hearing-handicapped patients this task may be accomplished early under amplification, using the patient's own hearing-aid if he uses one. Prior to cessation of the procedure, it must be accomplished routinely under normal voice production conditions, with the patient using his own aid if he will wear one but under no amplification otherwise, because this is closest to his daily listening conditions. The possibility of using stored signals recorded by various talkers is one to be considered so that the patient doesn't learn the idiosyncratic acoustic cues of a single voice in favor of more generally occurring cues of various voices.

Finally, the patient will have achieved some discrimination that can be expected to be less than adequate and he must learn to accept some significant rate of error in his routine listening. However, the therapist and the patient should both have an excellent idea of what sounds he tends to interconfuse (though patients who confuse /f/ for /s/ will not necessarily confuse /s/ for /f/). The therapist can then teach the patient what possible misidentifications he will experience, their likelihood—again based jointly on his particular problems and the relative importance (relative frequency of occurrence) of those in our language—and teach him to be distributional in approach when attempting to make sense out of the context he is receiving.

In each case, our model makes us realize that to maximize hit rates, we must accept some accompanying high false alarm rates. To say that another way, the more unwilling I am to misidentify an /f/ as an /s/, the less often I will be able to identify an /f/ as an /f/. One cannot understand conversations without risking error.

To review, then, if one finds himself with a patient who needs speech or hearing therapy, within the framework of our model, the need can be met by using any or all of the components. One can alter the dimension on which the information is processed with the idea that the distributions will have better separation with some new or partially new criterion variable. Alternatively, one can increase discriminability of the distributions in question on the original dimension. Finally, one can manipulate the criterion.

The Rational Criterion Hypothesis

Early in the section introducing the structure of the model, we mentioned the concept that clinicians can be expected to differ from one another because of varying experiential backgrounds. Our experiences— our memories—represent sets of accepted hypotheses or sets of expectations about the world, and these will not be identical from person to person. In spite of this individual variation, this presentation has assumed that the therapist's judgment is superior to that of the patient's; that the therapist's sets of distributions and sets of criteria are to be the standard for all sorts of judgment processes. Is this reasonable and if so, why?

The answer to the first part of this question is an obvious yes; the second part will be pursued in detail in Chapter 5, but to a lesser degree now. Our basic satisfaction with the competence of the therapist stems from a psychological starting assumption that the human being is relatively rational, and typically so about those things that occur most frequently. His rational behavior becomes preeminent as he experiences a state of affairs repeatedly, so that he builds up reliable distributions of variations in the state of affairs, about more important and less important positive and negative considerations in his payoff matrix, and about appropriate selection of criteria to optimize his payoff.

Does the therapist become progressively more rational in his use of the components of therapy leading to competence? Yes, if some few aspects of his training program orient him properly, and we will talk of this later. We will deal now only with certain of these things that have direct bearing on our present discussion. In general, if the therapist is well-trained in what are the appropriate observations to be used as a base for his decision axis and in how much weight to give to each type of observation, then as long as he experiences enough observations to build stable distributions, he will do so. In addition, he can, through his own trial and error, or through being so trained during his professional preparation, establish appropriate criteria for use in the clinical setting. The more opportunity to observe the clinician is afforded, once he is taught to observe, the better will be his perception of the distributional aspects of various speech and hearing qualities. The same experiences he uses to form stable observations will cause him to establish optimal criteria separating distributions because it is most economical to have optimal criteria. Deviating from the optimum in either direction yields an uneconomical payoff matrix that causes the clinician to self-correct. Repeated experience allows the exposure necessary to see his errors and correct them.

An extremely important concept is that precisely the same experience is open to the patient. He also should be considered as a rational processor in the sense that his present speech is economical for his perceptions of the distributional aspects of that speech, even though we, with our more realistic observational sets, consider it substandard, and for his criteria, which we consider less than optimally located. Given the payoff necessary to construct more appropriate decision axes—that is, some alteration of his environment so that he perceives it to be better to change than to continue his present speech—he will move to the new speech.

This is not to suggest that one must explain to the patient in these terms that speech is distributional, or that he must alter his decision axis.

Quite obviously, one can shape a patient's behavior without any understanding of the theory on his part or without even his knowledge that he is being manipulated. Consider the implication in the opposite case. When a patient does not alter his speech, it means he finds greater economy in maintaining the pattern than in altering it. It may be that his milieu so rewards him, perhaps unwittingly, that the therapist will have a fearsome fight to alter the situational payoff matrix. If such is the case, it becomes incumbent upon the therapist to provide a very high number of responses from the patient with high reinforcement for acceptable responses and a complete lack of reward for nonacceptable (present speech) responses.

A further implication is that often early therapy progresses because of what appears to be the importance to the patient of pleasing the therapist. This motivation is genuine clinical currency and it should be used by the therapist exactly as reward for clinical progress—and not for leaving Mommy without screaming, which should be treated as though it were simple expectation by the therapist. But for the long-range success of the patient, the importance of pleasing the therapist should be only a minimal contributor to the payoff matrix.

It is no easy task for the therapist to balance the advantage of having the patient willing to work hard to please him and his realization that a different payoff matrix must be constructed for the patient if the speech improvement is to be sustained.

THE PRINCIPLE OF REWARD-CONTINGENT BEHAVIOR

Fortunately, the principle formulated by Premack should serve to assist the therapist in this difficult procedure: "For any pair of responses the more probable one will reinforce the less probable one." [8] This principle means that if you want to elicit a behavior of low probability from the patient, make some high probability behavior contingent upon it. First you do what I want because it is followed by a little time for doing what you want. The examples that could be used to illustrate Premack's principle are so well-known, once pointed out, that we might wonder about the necessity of including them. Most of us have probably experienced the principle very early, when mother said, "Eat your Pablum and you can have some delicious whoosis." And we did, because whoosis was delicious and worth putting up with all the pap for. At this very moment many of us are probably reading a book we have to read to pass a course

[8] Premack, "Reinforcement Theory," *Nebraska Symposium on Motivation.*

so that we can do what we really would like to do. Our goal is to aid some people who have particular kinds of communication problems and need the kinds of help that only we can provide. So we put up with the reading and the studying and the performance necessary to pass the course, not particularly because we enjoy passing courses but because the less probable response of passing the course is reinforced by the opportunity to engage in therapy when we have done so.

Of course, most therapists have had an understanding of this principle prior to the formulation of it in this text (or by Premack), but the principle is of sufficient potential power as to bear both the telling and the repeating. Further discussion will be left for Chapter 5 because it is more appropriate to our consideration of the therapist than of the patient.

We have discussed the concept that the clinician is a rational processor of speech. He is rational because he is economical in his execution of repeated tasks insofar as he gradually constrains his strategies until he achieves a maximal payoff. His training provides him with the knowledge and understanding of what should be optimal payoff, and his training in observation gives him the tools for employing his knowledge.

The clinician can be presumed to have sufficient knowledge about the parameters of speech to achieve both the necessary spread and sharpening of distributions as well as the knowledge needed to predict the errors that will arise with various conditions limiting separation of distributions and the strategy and criteria to be used to maximize performance under these circumstances.

Measuring Change During Therapy

If we return for a moment to the representation of our model as a pair of overlapping distributions, the location of any criterion cut will divide the right-hand distribution into hits and misses and, at the same time, divide the left-hand distribution into false alarms and correct rejections. The hits and false alarms are those proportions of the two distributions to the right of the criterion cut and the misses and correct rejections are the proportion of the distributions to the left of the criterion cut. If we are willing to assume the normal distributions shown in Figure 21, then we can work backwards from a calculation of hits and false alarms to determine the location of the criterion cutoff in each distribution and, thereby, the distinctiveness of the two distributions as well.

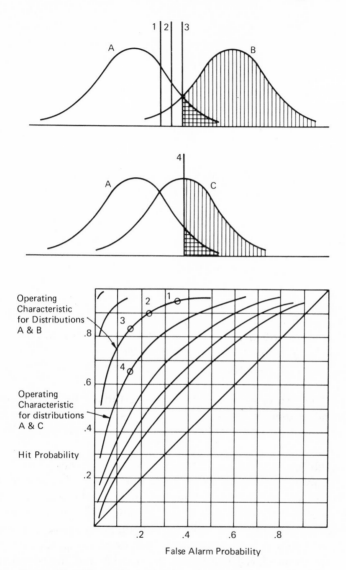

FIGURE 21. *Illustrative operating characteristics (oc) for distributions with varying magnitudes of discriminability and with varying criterion cutoffs.* (The curve labeled 321 in the lowest illustration represents the oc for the two distributions shown in the top illustration, and the three data points show the hit—false alarm likelihood ratios occurring by use of cutoffs 1, 2, and 3.)*
* The operating characteristic is the plot of the hit to false alarm relationship generated by passing a criterion cutoff through two normal distributions of equal variance (See Chapter Six for more complete explanation).

For any given task, organized in a closed-set paradigm, the clinician can plot his own hit and false alarm proportion, plot those of the patient, and use the comparison of the two to determine if the patient has adequate distribution distinctiveness and adequate cutoff location. In this way the therapist can separate problems in discrimination of the distributions from those relating to payoff matrix (criterion cutoff location). To see the particulars of such procedures, let us consider an example.

Consider therapy planning for a child producing routine $/\theta/$s substitutions. We can say that we must first determine if he hears the distinction in the speech of others. The therapist can produce, as an example, 400 nonsense syllables with $/s/$ and $/\theta/$ occurring equally often randomly in various phonemic syllable positions. The child chooses one or the other response each time, and we can calculate our result from these data. Let us choose $/s/$ as our signal (calculating on the basis of $/\theta/$ as the signal will derive exactly the same criterion cut and distributional distinctiveness so the choice is not critical). The proportion of $/s/$ signals correctly identified is our hit proportion (or hit rate); the proportion of $/\theta/$ signals misidentified as $/s/$ is the false-alarm proportion. Both hit and false-alarm proportions can now be converted to z scores of normal distributions and the distance between the means of the two distributions can be determined as a z-score distance.

The same experimental task can be performed by a group of children normal in their articulation ability and of the same age to yield an average normal separation and criterion cutoff location.

In addition, we can ask: Does the child have comparable or adequate discrimination for his own production of $/s/$ and $/\theta/$? So let us replicate the task but now have the child produce the nonsense syllable himself. After each production, both the child and the therapist make a decision as to whether the child's production was appropriate for the signal item. Again using $/s/$ as the signal item, the proportion of $/s/$ signals correctly produced constitutes the hit rate and the proportion of $/\theta/$ signals incorrectly produced constitutes the $/s/$ false-alarm rate. Note that a $/\theta/$ signal incorrectly produced means that the child was instructed to produce a $/\theta/$ but the therapist considers it an $/s/$, so that both hits and false alarms will probably show low proportions. The hits will be few because this is exactly the problem for which the child is in therapy, and the false alarms will be low because the child has substitution troubles only the other way (θ/s rather than s/θ). However, the low hit and false-alarm rates relate to criterion location, whereas our interest in this procedure is evaluating the discrimination of the child for his own productions relative to his discrimination for productions of other persons. We will obtain our desired information about his discrimination and need not concern ourselves with the occurrence of low hit and false-alarm rates.

Within this framework, if the patient's responses demonstrate that he has achieved the normal distinctiveness between distributions, as evaluated by his own performance, then therapy would be directed toward altering the patient's criterion cutoff. If the hit and false-alarm rates indicate that the patient is employing less than appropriate distribution distinctiveness, therapy would be directed toward this goal.

In the same manner, one can measure such aspects as: (1) the progress of therapy as the patient closes the gap by processing progressively more like the therapist; (2) the course of therapy, expressed as variation in rate from session to session: (3) the relationship of therapeutic procedure to the patient's progress; (4) therapists' efficiency with various kinds of pathologies (or some other, more appropriate, labeling scheme); (5) the patient's performance independent of his criterion.

Another reason for belaboring the point that the individual processes optimally for his payoff matrix is to pave the way for pointing up some significant implications for speech therapy and speech improvement procedures.

When a child demonstrates an articulatory disorder expressing a lack of distinctiveness on some significant decision axis or dimension, therapy should be structured to assist him in developing more comprehensive and contrastive speech-production distributions. He requires significant amounts of practice combined with rewards contingent upon his performing with progressively greater success in learning the distinction the therapist wants him to learn. Note that the assumption that he operates to a rational criterion indicates that when he has learned there is an important distinction, the learning coming about because the contrast clearly carries a reward that influences his payoff so that he is prepared to perform, and when he has sufficient exposure to the sets of observations, he will move to an appropriate criterion cutoff on his own volition. By that we mean that the patient will adopt the cost and value payoff matrix of the therapist when he has the knowledge of the therapist. There are techniques for such accomplishment—programmed therapy devices that are or can be automated—and these provide large numbers of exposures and can be adjusted for an appropriate payoff. It is comforting to find that, insofar as the success of such devices is now legion, the model predicts that this should be so.

Another observation can be made on the relationship between distributions and criteria. Given sufficient numbers of observations of speech as language—that is, in situations also yielding insight into culturally established payoff—if we adopt the rational criterion hypothesis, we seldom should find ourselves in the therapy situation wherein the goal is specifically to shift the criterion of the patient. Typically the patient's problem is distributional distinctiveness. He already knows the punishments and rewards of unsatisfactory or satisfactory speech. Infrequently a shift in cutoff may come about as a consequence of being exposed to a large number of observations from both distributions in question. Ordinarily, however, shifts in cutoff are not necessary nor do they occur. The occasions for which it would be desirable to train a client to shift his criterion are those in which the payoff matrix of the client differs from that of the typical person in the society.

Some few special classes of society constitute the major cases wherein the speech patterns of these groups have characteristics distinguishing them from that of the general society; for example, the ghetto population. A second major class encompasses those who cannot use the payoff matrix of the society effectively; for example, the profoundly handicapped in hearing. We have already discussed how one might increase the information available to the second group to alter their values and their distributions.

Our model should now make it obvious that, if one were to decide that it would be desirable to bring the speech patterns of the first group into consonance with those of the general society, the basic habilitation scheme should be directed first toward altering the costs and values of the group, then toward giving them significant exposure to the speech of the general population, and only later introducing the use of particular speech procedures.

Implications for Second Language Learning

There has been much interest in the past several years in an argument about how specific some portion of the central nervous system is in its genetic predisposition to the learning of language. One piece of evidence offered for the view that language is, to some degree, "prewired" is the presumed impossibility of an adult's learning a new language in which he could pass as a native speaker. The view expressed throughout this work is exactly contrary to such a stance. It suggests that an adult can learn a language for the first time and speak it indistinguishably from a native but to do so requires learning many tasks not typically accomplished in foreign language training.

Our typical learning procedures stress acquisition of a lexicon and the rules of grammar so that only these portions of language learning are stressed, rewarded, and mastered. What reveals the talker as a non-native is his use of phonetic and prosodic features that are not expected in the speech of natives and which thereby raise questions about the linguistic origins of the talker, alerting us to be still more careful in our processing of these small but potent cues. What the learner is relying upon while making such errors, is the wide latitude allowed such features in his native language as, for the most part, we are tolerant of great variability in such highly redundant aspects of the message. What he does not consider, however—and this is the key to his being unmasked as a non-native—is that the same distributional aspects, including the establishment and maintenance of criteria, apply to our perception of these "less important" components of the speech output as to the more important. The listener may be willing to accept any one of several prosodic patterns as appropriate to an utterance, including virtually infinite variation within the bounds of these patterns, but he will not accept without questioning himself as to what is wrong, any prosodic pattern outside that bounded set. Because the learner does not attend to minor but systematic constraints in prosodic patterning when learning a new language, he tends to concentrate upon lexical and grammatical considerations to the exclusion of these other cues that reveal his recent mastery. This is not to say that one could not learn all the attributes for speaking like a native were attention focused on them and were the learner given sufficient opportunity for large response output with feedback and reinforcement.

In the same way, middle-class American English is different from "ghetto" speech, and the same principles would need to be applied for an adult native talker of the latter to learn the former. The problem is not only one of specific vocabulary or of differences in precision of referents, but it also involves these finer cues to the social origins of the talker.

Therapy Processes, in Summary

We have defined the role of the therapist, if we pull together appropriate points scattered throughout our discussion of the therapy process, as comprising four areas:

1. The therapist must first control the environment in which therapy takes place. The control will involve commanding the physical

surroundings in which the interaction occurs, in that the therapist will determine the number and types of activities being carried on. Unsolicited and uncontrolled activities operate to the marked detriment of the process of eliciting and reinforcing desired responses by the patient and are antagonistic to the process of modifying interpersonal behavior.

Note that there are few restrictions we would impose on the physical characteristics of the environment. Windows overlooking locations of action that might be distracting must be avoided, but as long as the psychological isolation is preserved, virtually any location is open to use. Psychological isolation is a matter of definition and may vary from patient to patient, from pathology to pathology, and even from time to time in the same patient. But these very few considerations discussed above will allow the therapist to derive a criterion appropriate to this decision for each patient. The goal is to control the surroundings to inhibit the presence of distractors that might reduce the high work output necessary to effective therapy.

2. The therapist must present signals to the patient that are appropriate to the therapeutic goals, and that motivate the patient to attend and to respond. We have said that the therapist must provide signals rather than stimuli to the patient because we can describe a signal by defining its properties in any one of several ways. A stimulus, on the other hand, is that in a signal to which the responder attends, and we have no way of knowing what part of our signal this might be. Of course, what we will be attempting will be to get the patient to attend to the portions of the signal that are necessary for him to generate the desired response. We wish to shape his perception of the possible stimuli and we can do this by presenting signals and motivating him to attend to them and respond to them. As his responses move into some acceptable range, we can conclude that the stimulus parameters on which he has fixed agree with ours for the classes of signal delivered (that is, in the linguistic samples used, within the kinds of stress and intonation patterns used, and so forth). The goal is to shape the perceptions of the patient so that he attends to the important characteristics of the signal, so that the stimulus parameters he does use are those he should use.

3. Once the therapist has motivated the patient to respond to the signals soliciting his attention and response, the therapist must provide feedback to him. This feedback must assist the patient in defining the components of acceptable and nonacceptable signals so that he can internalize the sets of distributions made up of these responses, and so

that he can place an appropriate fence separating acceptable from non-acceptable responses (productions).

4. In addition to the preceding area and as an adjunct to it, the therapist must reinforce the acceptable responses from the patient in order to increase their frequency of occurrence in competition with the nonacceptable (former pattern) responses.

We seem to have sketched the ground rules for much of the therapeutic regime without trying to fill in all the details. There are a few additional points which may not be as obvious to the reader as most other conclusions and we shall try to deal with some of these. They are not presented in any particular order, and it should not be assumed that they are the most important points. They are merely some of those that seem relevant but not obvious.

First, if a major role of the therapist is to reinforce the patient's acceptable responses, he must have some perception of what the patient would consider a reinforcer. The most obvious way to get such information is to ask for it, so that one consideration in constructing an evaluative interview is the question of potential reinforcers.

Second, if a patient's unacceptable responses (speech productions) can be considered to have attained their output frequencies because they were previously reinforced, then the earlier any therapeutic regime is begun, the more easily one should be able to replace any unacceptable with an acceptable output. In public school therapy, the implication is clearly that of markedly increasing therapy efficiency (in ways we shall presently discuss) and achieving much more rapid caseload turnover. In such a problem as that of aberrant nonfluencies, as occur in the speech of stutterers, what may be required is a carefully thought-out program of sequential small changes in patient behavior, but the sooner the better.

Further, we can now again ask the question we posed previously: If you can accept only one additional patient, is it better to select a patient with a moderate voice problem or a mild stuttering? Such a question involves two considerations in its answer. The first concerns the implications of not remedying the problem. Will the continuing vocal insult introduce irreversible pathology? Will the mild stuttering induce other behavioral manifestations that engender a negative social reaction? The other consideration requires some thought by the therapist on the implications for each therapeutic regime of beginning now or holding off the commencement for a specified period of weeks or months. Our own previous analysis of the components that seem to control changes in behavior in human beings suggests that this second factor should be considered less important than the first, but some thought should be given to both.

Third, and this point has been made previously, therapeutic techniques must be evaluated by their relative abilities to generate response. The higher the output rate, the more effective the therapy and the therapist. We must begin to apply to our therapeutic procedures well established techniques designed to maximize both the economy and the effectiveness of therapy. Both goals require an objectification of the therapeutic process and the present suggestion provides the medium for beginning such a measurement. How much output does a therapy generate and how long does it take the patient to improve and be discharged?

Fourth, the therapist and his teacher must systematically attack the problem of the social considerations in the payoff matrix of good speech and hearing. At issue, of course, is the patient's perception of the price he pays for his own speech or hearing problems, which constitutes a significant factor both in the patient's motivations and the likelihood that clinical treatment will change his daily speech.

Perhaps early observation activities for the therapist-in-training will help provide the basis for understanding many of the motivations of individuals in situations of communication stress. While it may be difficult to structure the kinds of observations and interactions the student needs during his training if he is to become sensitive to patients' perceptions of their own communication problems, we must make progress in our understanding of the motivations of patients if we are to use them.

Our goal in therapy is to optimize some aspects of the behavior of the patient. We will try to do this with a minimum of clinical time and energy, consistent with having the patient accomplish the change in his daily communication habits. Probably the key to the patient's progress in therapy and his ultimate adequacy in communication is our own particular ability to understand and use the communication payoff matrix held by the patient.

FIVE

Training

It may seem inappropriate to have a section on training, but the aim of this chapter is consistent with the remainder of the text. Our goal is to evaluate the use of a model for clinical decisions and, in this chapter, to ask what the application of the model to areas of our own training might reveal as guiding principles to be learned and as informational content necessary to competent clinical practice.

Many aspects of training provide necessary tools for the professional person which need not be sequenced. In this category we can place such skills as professional personal conduct, interchanging information with coprofessionals, mastering skillful use of tests and materials, and the like. Other aspects of professional training do seem to operate on an internal logic that may dictate that some one of a very few available sequences be used in mastering the material. Examples include the sequencing of early observation experiences to be description, perception and inference-making, as one deals with information gathering and information synthesizing. An additional example, perhaps not so compelling, is observation of normal processes, then direct observation of variables open to pathological distortions of interest in speech and hearing, and subsequently, observation of variables influencing conditions of interest in speech and hearing.

Part of what is important in such a sequence is learning what to observe as well as how to observe. Both of these aspects of observation are based in skills, to be learned, of classification and categorization. We must learn which potential criteria are to be accentuated and which are to be attentuated. These in turn involve goal evaluation, as the utility of the criterion is defined by its assistance toward pursuit of the goal. It is this sort of internal logic that serves to organize the experiences made available to the student. He must learn to observe long before he can participate in goal planning and evaluation, but he will learn appropriate observation skills only if his supervisor has already structured their relationship to the goals. By the same token, the student will probably have difficulty throughout all of his training, and perhaps all of his career, if he tries to master goal planning and evaluation without having mastered earlier observation skills.

Therefore the student, observing for purposes of understanding clinical dyadic interactions, must observe with full understanding of the goals of the interaction even though he is not yet sufficiently experienced to engage in goal planning activities. His knowledge of the goals of the session structures his observation—categorization skills. Much of this discussion revolves on observation experiences because of their central importance to professional preparation. Of the large number of skills we must learn in the course of achieving adequate clinical performance, a high proportion seem to be communicated only through the medium of clinical practice. Some of these we seem able to master by participation in simulations of various types, others require that we be allowed to "see for ourselves" while under the guidance of assisting master clinicians. But our introduction to all of these as well as other skills and experiences comes through the medium of clinical observation, and we shall give our early attention to observation as a training procedure.

First, let the reader remind himself that observing a process does not necessarily give insight into the goals of the process, a point we have made, but also that observing behavioral patterns under modification does not necessarily give any clues into why these particular patterns were chosen for modification.

Why might one observe, and for what purposes?

1. To experience both the occurrence of pathology and its characteristics and the occurrence of normal and its characteristics
2. To observe the occurrence of inferred cause-effect relationships
3. To attempt and experience prediction of behavior, which involves gaining insights into motivations
4. Given a model for the information necessary to an evaluation, to observe the acquisition of information for evaluation
5. To observe application of therapeutic procedures, as long as the observer has been oriented to the need for a patient-centered rather than a clinician-centered or technique-centered therapy.
6. To observe the application of professional judgments, in the absence of personal value judgment, as part of the professional attitude

Items 2–6 above would all represent different observation experiences if the observer were familiar with information concerning the patient rather than were he uninformed.

To appreciate further uses to be made of observation experiences, we need only consider some additional skills necessary to the independent professional:

1. Learn inference-making and decision-making processes
2. Learn professional demeanor and attitudes
3. Develop professional empathy (we will beg the question of whether it can be learned as an adult)
4. Learn professional communication, both oral and written, and interchange of information, predictions, speculations, and so forth, with co-professionals
5. Learn standard institutional operating procedures

Observation experiences can be useful in forwarding acquisition of each of these skills. By the same token, we could have structured much of this discussion in terms of group meetings and their uses, or therapy simulations, evaluation simulations, and the like.

The student might find it convenient to organize his observation experiences by age level of patients. Probably considerations of patient motivation and patient behavior modification are more easily organized this way than by any other single characteristic. However, this organizing scheme can be expected to be economical only for observation experiences in which the observer is interested in patient classification rather than procedure classification. Because observation should play such a central role in student training, we will address ourselves to some general considerations to which we should attend in thinking about such experiences.

The Role of Observation in Training

As a corollary to reaching any decisions about others, the clinician must learn to separate his decisions from his observations. He must learn to observe and he must learn to describe the observation. We can use the model for therapy we have already described to focus on this area of training. Discovering whether a student can describe and training him to do so requires that the student supply output and that a clinician evaluate it and supply feedback, with reinforcement for appropriate responses.

One can do this by requiring that the student engage in X hours observing therapy—and only therapy, for reasons shortly to be described —and submit reports of these observations. The student may or may not be allowed to draw inferences from his observations but, if so, they should be separated in his text and labeled as such. The student *must* have such observations returned promptly, rigorously corrected and graded. He should be required to resubmit any observations that are contaminated by inference. Alternatively or additionally, the student can be assigned to observe evaluations undertaken by master clinicians (never clinicians in training) and can be expected to report in the clinical conference on his observations of particular portions of the evaluation; for example, the patient's spontaneous speech, or the patient's reactions to various portions of structured testing procedures. In these clinical conferences, there can be immediate feedback in the event the student slips from an observation to an inference mode of performance, and there can be immediate reinforcement for appropriate performance, and so forth.

EVALUATING OBSERVATIONS

This type of student participation in clinical conferences has the additional advantage that the student learns to place a greater value on some observations than others, so he begins to learn the importance of various components in constructing a decision axis. That is, he properly learns the difference between an observation and an inference from some observation(s). But he also has the advantage of finding himself in a circumstance in which he can draw tentative conclusions from his observations and derive feedback about these. Note that all three tasks—learning to observe, to draw inferences from observations, and to distinguish one from the other—are conducted in a social setting having significant reinforcing properties for the student.

A CAUTION ON OBSERVATION OPPORTUNITIES

One other condition accrues to the clinical conference. We have already suggested that the student needs many exposures to therapy sessions so that he can derive ideas of how various therapies are conducted, how effective various therapeutic procedures are with various patients, how some therapy styles seem to fit one patient—therapist interaction but not another, and so forth. We have also previously suggested that the student needs many exposures to persons with normal speech or hearing and these observations can probably be carried on individually in the community by assignment once the student has reached some pre-established level of observation ability (except for some selected observations to be discussed).

These types of experience are designed to assist the student in building distributions of observations, in one case for persons already found to be pathological, in the other case for persons within the normal range. Neither type of experience presents the student with a problem of defining criteria (locating fences) so neither is contaminated by the student's immaturity in deriving such judgments. However, the clinical evaluation is a different type of experience and must be viewed as such.

In the clinical evaluation, the student finds himself faced with the requirement of making a decision about the presence or absence of non-normal speech or hearing, with all the addenda following such a decision. This quite obviously is a matter concerning the placement of criteria about which the student has little experience and he tends to find himself accepting the criteria of his older classmates with their seemingly superior knowledge and insight. It is therefore particularly important that the student's exposure early in his program be only to evaluations done by experienced clinicians if he is to be allowed any exposure at all. As stated above, it is advantageous for the student to be allowed to participate in clinical evaluations and the conferences that follow, but his role should be restricted to aspects of an observational nature or, at most, to primitive inferences from his observations. The additional yield to the student will be the opportunity to experience the construction of a decision about the patient, which carries with it significant inferences about the components of the clinical decision axis.

THE CAUTION ON OBSERVATION RESTATED

The majority of training programs in our discipline provide observation experiences of evaluation and diagnosis as well as observation of therapy for potential future clinicians early in their training. This exposure serves both as a recruiting device for the profession and as a medium for maintaining the interest of the student before he comes to personal clinical exposure. In addition, observation opportunities serve a positive function for the student in increasing the size of the sample he uses to estimate distributions of various defects. It should be kept in mind, however, that a program does a disservice to the stu-

dent if it gives him repeated exposures to other students attempting
to dichotomize patients on normal/pathological continua (that is, evaluate patients) when neither the student examiner nor the observer has
sufficiently detailed experience to place a valid clinical criterion on the
continuum. Observation of these labeling events should come late in
the student's training and preferably only by exposure to master clinicians. Early academic knowledge and observation should be available
only for therapy, because observation of previously (and, presumably,
expertly) evaluated patients allows the professional-in-training to build
reasonable distributions and appropriate fences. After the student has
had frequent exposure to persons in therapy and has learned the ways
in which the speech, voice or language differs from that of the normal,
then exposure to a master examining clinician helps the budding professional to locate an appropriate criterion for the disorder under
evaluation.

EXPANDING OBSERVATION OPPORTUNITIES

Let us revert to a point glanced over earlier. We indicated that a
student requires significant observation experiences with persons in both
normal and pathological distributions. If the caseload of the training
institution is sufficiently large and carefully constituted, most observations necessary to dimensionalizing the pathological population can be
obtained directly in the speech and hearing center. For most college
students, however, there are few opportunities to observe a broad spectrum of the normal population, particularly the two ends of the age
range. One way of achieving such exposure for the student is to assign
him routine responsibilities in a normal nursery school as well as in a
home for the aged. Most college communities have the former, and
progressively more of the latter are coming into existence as developers
of such institutions begin to appreciate the social and cultural advantages of any campus. Requiring public school teaching experience is
a less satisfactory way of obtaining the pediatric exposure for prospective
teachers or even for those clinicians not preparing for school positions,
because schools tend to be organized as more formal structures and
children in school probably show a more constrained behavior than do
populations of the nursery or the home for the aged.

STORED OBSERVATION OPPORTUNITIES

An alternative, or supplement, to all of the above types of exposure
designed to facilitate the formation of distributions by the student is

the extensive use of audio and video tapes from libraries maintained by the individual college speech and hearing centers. An even more desirable suggestion is to have a scientific committee of the American Speech and Hearing Association write a recommended standard for both audio and video recording and reproduction with a goal of achieving national compatibility in equipment. We could then utilize one another's libraries of tapes, or establish tape banks with dubbing facilities for inexpensive reproduction and distribution. Following shortly thereafter, it should be possible to construct sets of equivalent items for a video-taped examination given to certify clinicians in evaluation procedures, in construction of therapy prescriptions, and like matters.

The early steps toward building such "standard" tapes were undertaken when D. Sherman and her colleagues began to scale various pathologies in speech.[1] Her approaches to achieving national uniformity of judgments did not meet with acceptance by most college teachers of clinicians so that now, approximately two decades later, we still show variance, one to another, in our clinical decisions (I call your moderate voice cases mild and you call my mild articulation problems normal.) The experimental procedures outlined by Sherman still provide the medium and necessary rigor for constructing scales of various magnitudes of pathologies, should researchers decide that such endeavors are worthy of new beginnings.

In addition to audio and video tapes to scale and teach magnitude of pathology, one can utilize this same medium to build a store of experiences with various therapeutic procedures. One can, by routine video recording and on-line or delayed appraisal, build a significant collection of therapist-patient interactions. One can sequence tapes presenting changes in patient response output with various therapeutic approaches, and this can be done for appraising the therapy or the therapist or both. Such tapes and such procedures could also provide an integral part of training sub-professionals, an issue discussed in succeeding sections.

It seems then that we should consider use of tape banks to increase the observation opportunities and experiences of our students and our future technician-trainees in evaluation, in building programs of ther-

[1] D. Sherman, "Clinical and Experimental Use of the Iowa Scale of Severity of Stuttering, "*Journal of Speech and Hearing Disorders,* 17 (1952), 316–320; and among others, D. Sherman and C. E. Moodie, "Four Psychological Scaling Methods Applied to Articulation Defectiveness," *Journal of Speech and Hearing Disorders,* 20 (1955), 352–358.

apy, in teaching contingency management, in observation of normal communication (particularly in the young and the old), and so forth. We should only add that probably subprofessional technicians would be restricted in their duties to specific types and classes of therapy so that many such tapes might illustrate quite similar clinical phenomena but where individual tapes were oriented toward different classes of technicians.

Quantification in Therapy, Therapists, and Would-be Therapists

If you as a student are a rational processor, as is your supervising clinician, and you and he do not agree in labeling some sample of speech, then you have not mastered the knowledge or gained the spectrum of clinical experience necessary to the construction of the appropriate decision axis. But whatever the reason for your inadequate performance, we hypothesize that you and he should reach the same decision if you process a necessary minimum of appropriate information and weight it properly. When you do not reach the same conclusion, it must be that you as a student are not using the appropriate information or you are poorly weighting some portion(s) of it. Your training therefore is inadequate for the speech or hearing problem under consideration at the time. In plain terms, this hypothesis directs the construction of objectively recorded and scaled samples to evaluate many aspects of clinical preparation. The growing competence of the student can be appraised by his performance using the decision axis, distributions, and criteria of the master clinicians with whom he is training. And, in like manner, we can require that he engage in various labeling tasks that can be designed to display the magnitude of agreement of his perceptions and those of his teachers. This is not different from the type of testing to which college undergraduates are routinely subjected, but we are herein asserting that it is possible to quantify the value-judgment processes underlying clinical decisions so that these could be objectified rather than left to the subjective insights (and biases) of the clinical supervisor.

In-Service Training Programs

All the trends projected above require that we pay some attention to updating the skills of clinicians currently in the field, as well as the orientation and areas of competence of those responsible for training future clinical personnel. Is there some priority that can be assigned to the various new dimensions of knowledge that must be mastered so that we can conduct in-service training programs that are both useful and economical? Such programs or seminars should revolve around four major foci. The first of these would be decision theory. This would be followed by development of specific procedures for learning and using behavioral engineering. The third would be systematic exposure of these workshop participants to normal communication experiences of all types, involving persons of all age groups with which the clinician would be working. The fourth and most difficult portion would attempt to teach programming techniques to our seminar group.

This fourth portion is most difficult because, like many other aspects of the teaching process, good programming is a highly creative art. Good therapy of any sort is an equally creative art, and we have devoted most of this book to distinguishing those portions of it that represent a skill and can be taught from those portions that are only mysteriously acquired. Ultimately, this means that some people will do most of our programming, and individual therapists will only minimally alter the sequencing though they will exert original and continuing control over the timing, the type and frequency of reinforcement, the choice of specific program, and so forth. However, any clinicians who will utilize such procedures should have some exposure to their construction. As a still more selfish motive, we will have to keep a sharp lookout for persons who do show such creative skills so that they can be enticed into building programs for use by all of us.

THE TRAINER

One final aspect of training must be dealt with—the role of the trainer. Only recently has there been significant interest, other than infrequent papers or convention presentations, in defining the role of supervision in clinical training and, more explicitly, in attempting to detail the activities of clinicians-in-training to open them to evaluation by the supervisor. Any book such as this one, which lays stress on supervised observation, on the close interaction of supervisor and student, and on the necessity that the student master the clinical skills of the supervisor, assumes some obligation to illuminate the process of supervision. We shall attempt to do so, in spite of the lack of assistance from the literature in speech and hearing. Even if we go to writings in other fields, we cannot have great confidence in present models because there have been no evaluations undertaken to determine whether or not an adapted model will work for us.

In spite of this, we will propose a model adapted from the field of teacher education. Our placing it in the chapter on training rather than the chapter on research is premature. Nevertheless, we present the model to give the student some grasp of the goals and structure of supervision. The model from which we have extrapolated this current system is one developed by H. Schalock [2] and freely adapted from his in *Mirrors for Behavior,* Vol. 12, 1970, to meet our professional purposes.

The model focuses upon the clinical dyad of the clinician–patient interaction. With a minor change in labels, it could be applied to various other two-person interactions and, in particular, we have in mind the supervisor with the clinician. An in-service training program for supervisors could use the same structure to have supervisors criticize each other in genuine or simulated supervision interactions.

The goals of any supervisory process are to bring the traits of the clinician's behavior to his own attention and to have the supervisor evaluate these traits by some means that the clinician himself can internalize as guides for his future behavior. Therefore, our model builds upon what we have repeatedly called the basic learning paradigm: the patient has engaged in some behavior motivated by the clinician's activities. The clinician must evaluate this performance on the part of the patient and provide some positive or negative evaluation as feedback.

Each message from the clinician to the patient will be considered as a distinct unit for appraisal, where a message is a single coherent communication or *move.* [3] A four-way appraisal system might employ these categories: (a) *Focus;* (b) *Substantive Content;* (c) *Clinical Operations;* and (d) *Affective Quality.* Each category will be developed

[2] H. Del Schalock, Clark Smith and Frances Vogel, "An Overview of the TEACHING RESEARCH System for the Description of Teaching Behavior in Context," in *Mirrors for Behavior: An Anthology of Classroom Observation Instruments,* Anita Simon and E. Gil Boyer, eds., Vol. 12, 1970.

[3] *Moves* are units of interaction initiated by the therapist or the supervisor to motivate some response behavior from the patient or subject. A *tactic* of interaction might be to precipitate performance by initiating an inquiry, whereas asking the particular question (for example, a verification question) would be a move.

in some detail but the last two require and will receive greater con-
centration than the first two.

Focus: We will appraise in detail only messages specifically directed
toward influencing either the attitudes or the performance of the patient
as concerns his own speech, hearing or language. To these ends, we
direct the attention of the supervisor first to the question of the focus
of the interaction. The supervisor must decide whether the interaction
is focused toward patient's *performance* or his *attitudes;* whether it is
misfocused on some behavior (s) not associated with the patient's speech,
language or hearing (and, perhaps, not appropriately a concern of the
therapist) ; or whether the interaction is unfocused.

Attention to the *attitudes* of the patient can be examined in detail,
by categorizing the particular attitudes under consideration as focusing
on (1) his attitudes toward himself and his own personal characteristics;
(2) his attitudes toward his own speech in its immediate or general
characteristics; (3) his attitudes toward the receiver of the communication, in general or as refers to the therapist; and (4) his attitudes
toward the underlying communication in content or intent.

Certainly we can agree that many interactions of clinician and
patient may influence the patient's performance, but our further evaluation of the clinical interaction and clinicians will be limited only to
behavior focused on the clinical *performance* of the patient. If the
supervisor determines that much of the transaction being observed is
improperly focused, then he might care to evaluate its affective quality,
but presumably he would choose not to deal with its content or procedures.

Given appropriate focus, we address three additional questions:

What *substantive content* does it contain?
What *clinical operations* does it represent?
What *affective qualities* does it contain?

To understand our expansion of these three questions, consider the
task of the patient. (1) He must obtain and process information about
his present and his expected speech or hearing behavior. (2) He must
test whether he has control over this information by performing in
relation to it. (3) He must receive feedback from the process.

Substantive Content: Evaluation in this category can be equated
with evaluative procedures used for our basic model, and follows from
prior discussion:

1. Does the content involve the underlying decision variable?
2. Does the content involve either or both means of the distributions?
3. Does the content involve either or both the variances of the distributions?
4. Does the content involve the patient's criterion space or cutoff location?

To deal in more detail with considerations of setting goals for therapy and achieving these goals, we would have to repeat much from earlier chapters. We will not, therefore, discuss the merit of a 1. content relative to a 2. content, expecting that the labeling of a clinical communication, from therapist to patient, as a 1. or a 4. objectifies it sufficiently to permit a value judgment of appropriateness.

Presumably, every clinician must become familiar with a wide variety of specific clinical levers potentially useful with a variety of patients. The more of these the clinician has available for routine use, the more likely he is to pick those most beneficial to the individual patient—that is, the more patient-centered the therapy is likely to be. The supervisor must distinguish many varieties of clinical messages and we have tried to catalog a wide variety.

The dimension of affective quality is structured to reflect necessary stages of therapeutic affect. We have spoken of the necessity that the clinician gradually alter the payoff of the patient from achievement by pleasing the clinician to achievement by pleasing a more general society, and we have tried to construct dimensions reflecting the necessary transitions.

Clinical Operations: These can be classified as follows:

1. Exposing the patient to information, extending his knowledge, increasing his awareness, and so forth, as long as the message contains no qualities that would lead to its being considered an evaluation of patient performance
2. Precipitating performance by the patient, broadly accompanied by inquiry or demand
3. Evaluating performance of the patient by assigning qualities of goodness/badness, and the like

Each of the clinical operations can be conducted by using various *tactics:*

1. Tactics: exposition, illustration, demonstration

2. Tactics: inquiry, direction
3. Tactics: signals, words, objects

Finally, we can consider that each clinical tactic can be accomplished by various *moves,* as in the following chart:

EXPOSURE TO INFORMATION

The Tactic of Exposition
   —describe that which is being considered
   —conceptualize that which is being considered
   —explain that which is being considered
   —evaluate that which is being considered

The Tactic of Illustration
   —provide positive examples of the state being considered
   —provide negative examples of the state being considered
   —provide an abstract model of the state being considered
   —provide a pictorial model of the state being considered
   —provide a representative model of the state being considered
—provide a real-life model of the state being considered.

The Tactic of Demonstration
   —provide a laboratory or simulated demonstration of the process
     or state being considered
   —provide a real-life demonstration of the process or state being
     considered

PRECIPITATION OF PERFORMANCE

Inquiry
   —conditional questions
   —verification questions
   —relational questions
   —implication questions

Direction
   —by suggestion
   —straightforward, accompanied by a cushion
   —straightforward, accompanied by an explanation
   —straightforward and without qualification

EVALUATION OF PERFORMANCE

Signals
   —tending
   —low-power signals
   —high-power signals

Words
   —by suggestion

—straightforward, accompanied by a cushion
—straightforward, accompanied by an explanation
—straightforward and without qualification

Objects
—low-power objects
—high-power objects

Using the structure proposed above, the supervisor can make a "running" evaluation of the clinical interaction as flowing from the clinician, and help the clinician to appreciate alternative moves, tactics, and so forth, that might assist him and his patient.

Affective Quality: The final question to which the supervisor addresses himself is that of the Affective Quality of the interaction. We will deal with the tone of the interaction by assigning one of three values to its emotional quality and further, splitting each dimension of our trichotomy again into three:

1. Warmth, interest, exuberance
2. Distance, aloofness
3. Upset, concern

For each of these quality sets, we assign a *zero* value to affective quality which is judged as being appropriate to the situation and the clinician under observation. For category 1, a + indicates somewhat more positive feeling than is appropriate, a + + indicates far more positive feeling than is appropriate.

For category 2, a / indicates somewhat more distance than is appropriate, a // indicates far more distance or aloofness than is appropriate.

For category 3, a — indicates the clinician expresses somewhat more upset or concern than is appropriate, a — — indicates far more concern or upset than is appropriate.

The clinician must begin by rewarding achievement and must continue to do so and, therefore, 1 has a positive value. There may be appearances of + + ratings in early therapy so that the patient works for this clinical currency, but there should not be a great number at any time. Even these few + + ratings should reduce in frequency during later therapy, as should + ratings, and therapy nearing termination should show few ratings other than 0 as 1 responses.

The second variable in affective quality expresses the supervisor's appraisal of the gradual removal of the clinician as the source of reward for the patient. A slowly increasing distance must be injected into the clinical dyad and, on the average, the major concern of the supervisor will be to insure that the rate is appropriate to both patient and clinician.

The final variable is presumed to be of equal importance in early experiences of a therapist-in-training because it can be expected that the therapist will often deliver an appropriately focused message that does not energize the behavior he is seeking. His concern with himself and his therapeutic approach may be misinterpreted by the patient as being a concern and negative evaluation on the patient's own performance, and may have deleterious effects on the therapy dyad. The evaluation of upset or concern is specified in an effort to keep the clinician aware of the importance of this aspect of his own reaction system.

Presumably, the clinician found to be markedly deviant when in his zero mode (in his typical behavior) should be removed from clinical interactions with patients until he can learn more temperate habits in professional circumstances.

One additional set of variables should be gauged by the supervisor, but these will receive only a single judgment for the entire observation session. Three distinct judgments having to do with the quality of the dyadic interaction are considered. First, is the interaction analogous to that between teacher and pupil, wherein the teacher alters the behavior or attitudes of the pupil without significant personal change occurring in himself? Or, is the interaction analogous to the psychotherapeutic dyad wherein both patient and therapist undergo significant change? Does the interaction represent a teacher/psychotherapist model?

Second, is the quality of the dyad established by the clinician or the patient or mutually by their interaction? For purposes of making the judgment, one asks the questions: Does the clinician control the quality of the interaction, does the patient do so, or is it established by their joint actions?

Finally, can the behavior of the clinician, in a bipolar characterization, be considered to be active or passive?

One final point might be usefully made about both supervision and general clinical training. The goal of the supervisor should always be to sharpen the clinician's perceptions, and thereby the clinician's behavior, in the clinical dyad. The clinician will provide some output for the supervisor by interacting with the patient, but the supervisor must both evaluate and transmit some feedback, with minimal delay, to the clinician. If the training location has the use of a video-tape recorder/reproducer, the clinician-in-training can be given the same evaluation form that his supervisor might use and be asked to criticise a video taping of his own clinical interaction with a patient, but the influence of such a procedure, while it might be great, should not be expected to be the same as the influence of immediate feedback from his supervisor while he still is in the grip of his immediately previous clinical session.

As of the time of this writing, there is already a requirement by the American Boards of Examiners in Speech Pathology and Audiology (the certifying agency for national certification in speech or hearing) that clinical experience be obtained under the direct supervision of someone certified as clinically competent. The implementation of this requirement places many more of us in a supervisory capacity than previously. Any significant evolution of the profession in the direction of using sub-professional technicians will further increase the proportion of professionals doing supervision of some sort. In-service training in supervision may become one of the most pressing needs we have and some public discussion and interchange of ideas and suggestions would be helpful to us all.

Needed Additional Components of Professional Training

STATISTICAL DECISION THEORY

Two requisites for the training of any kind of clinicians are imperative. They are statistical decision theory and behavioral management. Without question, any person attempting to engage in modifying interpersonal behavior requires some introduction to statistical decision theory. Interestingly enough, the programs in the major universities, as well as in most other programs graduating more than a few students a year, all seem to require their students to have exposure to at least one course in statistical techniques. This, we can assume, is to help the student read and understand the research literature in, or appropriate to, his field. But the decision theory that would supply the structure for understanding and interpreting these same statistics is seldom offered, if one can believe the catalog course descriptions. Further, we can probably make a strong case for the position that understanding general decision processes in situations of probabilistic information is significantly more important than facility in manipulating various statistics. But the overall point to be stressed is that clinicians find themselves having to alter decision behaviors in their patients to insure that the patients improve in communicative ability. It would seem that this should be most easily accomplished if the therapist has some good idea of how human beings make decisions, and how they are open to being altered once made, and statistical decision theory provides a good and relatively simple model of such a process.

BEHAVIORAL ENGINEERING

The area of preparation, in addition to decision theory, that should be requisite to clinical participation—that is fundamental to understanding the art of modifying interpersonal behavior—is that of behavioral engineering through controlling stimuli and managing reinforcement contingencies. The importance of this area of study has been mentioned repeatedly in the course of presenting our model of clinical processes. Perhaps the reader, like many of my colleagues, feels that these procedures do not have the behavior-modification power asserted for them for *any* speech or hearing problem, on the average, and that they have virtually no utility at all for remedying many specific speech or hearing problems. This question can be left open for empirical determination by researchers and clinicians in the field. We need only ask that these kinds of procedure receive adequate trial in open and balanced competition and that the results of these experiments be published in our professional journals. The areas of speech and hearing remediation for which these newer procedures have greater utility than the more classic therapeutic protocols will be revealed by such experimentation, and clinicians will be able to choose their own therapeutic procedures as they have always done.

It must be noted, however, that the employment of a corps of technicians has some promise of success only if we can markedly tighten the structure of the therapist-patient interaction. We cannot train nor expect to achieve such insights in our technicians as are fundamental to present remedial techniques within the duration and depth of training they will probably receive. Therefore, if we do not undertake the necessary explorations and research to learn techniques of modifying behavior and to explore their utility for all areas of speech and hearing, we will find ourselves with the progressively greater problem of trying to meet the demands made upon the profession with techniques and personnel not capable of being stretched that far. Our society places continually greater stress upon communication skills in an increasingly larger percentage of the society, and our training programs do not keep up with the increasing demand nor can they even try to fill present demands. We must make dramatic advances in the economy of our therapies; and the behavioral management approaches of Holland & Skinner,[4] Homme,[5] and Garrett & the Riggs'[6] offer what may be the best available route for these dramatic changes.

[4] Holland and Skinner, *Analysis of Behavior: Programmed Instruction.*
[5] Homme, "Contiguity Theory and Contingency Management" *The Psychological Record,* 16, 233–241.
[6] Garrett, *Speech and Language Therapy Under an Automated Stimulus Control System;* and among others, K. E. and J. C. Rigg, *Behavioral Engineering: Adaptation of Emotional Behavior.* Report 69–001, Communication Research Lab, Department of Speech, New Mexico State University, January 1969.

SIX

Research

The primary purpose of this chapter on research is to deal with the acquisition of data necessary to the application of this or alternative models. We have sketched procedures for altering our training that require many kinds of knowledge not currently available. We have suggested techniques for evaluating progress in therapy also requiring new materials. In addition, we have presented specific suggestions for research in previous sections and these are gathered together and restated in following sections.

The various suggestions for research are categorized and presented in six sections: personnel, speech characteristics, speech attitudes, therapy, training, and multicategory phenomena and their relations. All of the studies suggested are seen as necessary to application of our general clinical model or arising from evaluation of the model. All involve the process of interpersonal communication and modifying interpersonal behavior. It is appropriate, therefore, that we open this chapter with a more careful consideration of this very process of speech communication and we will proceed to do so by evaluating a model. It should rapidly become obvious that the speech communication model has the same heritage as our clinical model; we introduce this alternative because it alters our focus from clinical strategies to interpersonal communication, per se.

A Model of Speech Communication

The communication act can be characterized as involving five highly interdependent elements, as seen in the following schema, and the entire system is encompassed in the question: "Who says what to whom in what situation and for what purpose?

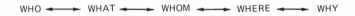

WHO ◄────► WHAT ◄────► WHOM ◄────► WHERE ◄────► WHY

FIGURE 22. *Components of human communication.*

While this block schema includes all that is necessary for specifying the communication act, it is not formed so as to be open to experimental investigation. To facilitate research, the schema must be expanded and couched in somewhat more operational terms. For this purpose, one can adopt and expand the very powerful model for communication proposed by Shannon,[1] and expanded most insightfully by Tanner.[2] The present schema includes additional modification to highlight some prospective sources of experimental interest.

The expanded model includes a communication chain of schematized components, plus noise source(s) which can be inserted in various locations. The noise perturbation can enter the system at any locus or loci and serves, upon introduction, to obscure the characteristics of the message, thereby reducing the probability that the communication will be successful.[3]

Several assertions are implicit in this model and these will be considered in turn, without consideration of priority or relative importance.

1. *Message ensembles* comprise all possible messages that can be generated by the *speaker* and, in the general case, are infinite in number in several ways. One can generate an infinity of sentences, an infinite set of meaningful sentences, or an infinite set of sentence fragments.

---

[1] C. E. Shannon, "The Mathematical Theory of Communication," in C. E. Shannon and W. Weaver, *The Mathematical Theory of Communication* (Urbana: University of Illinois Press, 1964).

[2] W. P. Tanner, Jr., "Physiological Implications of Psychophysical Data," in J. A. Swets, ed., *Signal Detection and Recognition in Human Observers* (New York: Wiley, 1964). Adapted from Tanner, in Swets, 1964, with permission.

[3] Successful communication means that the receiver responds in the manner desired by the speaker. One need not require, however, that the receiver initiate a response message to the speaker; instead, one can have the receiver transmit a message to the experimenter. In that case one has a measure of the first transmission (speaker to receiver) if and only if the second transmission (receiver to experimenter) does not involve any deterioration.

The transmission can be evaluated directly by measuring the amount of reduction in uncertainty following the presentation of the signal from the uncertainty in the receiver about the content of the message prior to its transmission. For details, see W. R. Garner, *Uncertainty and Structure as Psychological Concepts* (New York: Wiley, 1962).

One can take any single sentence or fragment and expand its communicated message by altering aspects of its phonology. Still further, one can alter its communicative content, not by altering its grammar or its phonology, but by altering the situation in which it is used—the social milieu, or the semantic environment, or the receiver to whom it is addressed.

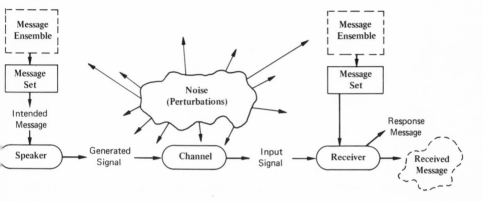

FIGURE 23. *Block diagram of one-way communication.*

2. While it is obvious that a *speaker* has the competence to generate an infinitude of messages, virtually any specific real-life communication situation so constrains his behavior that he, in fact, samples from only a finite *Message Set*. One simply does not communicate certain things to certain people (or, perhaps, to any person) in certain situations. So while the message ensemble comprises an infinite set, the message set is highly limited and finite.

In the sense that the task could be done if one were convinced it would yield a return commensurate with the effort, detailing the total set of messages in the set for some given communication situation is merely an engineering problem; the task is possible, the techniques are available, and the only question that need arise is whether the job is worth doing.

3. The *Intended Message* and the *Generated Signal* need not be identical. This is obvious when friends communicate privileged information in a coded form during the course of an open conversation in the presence of others, not privy to the shared experiences. The friend has different expectations than the other listeners and the result is different information being obtained from the same spoken message by the two types of receivers.

It may be less obvious, though equally true, when one listens to the query "Vest?" from a stranger. If this question arises when the receiver is standing in a clothing store, he will probably decide the intended message is, "Where can I buy a vest?", and he will direct the speaker to the location in the store wherein the item is displayed. If, however, the question arises when the receiver is standing on a street corner, he will probably decide that the intended message was, "Which way is West?", and he will respond accordingly, being highly directionally oriented. In each case, the receiver treats the communication by working through the signal to the intended message, though the mapping from the one to the other is different in the two examples, and the receipt of the generated signal and the determination of the correct intended message are both probabilistic.

It is prudent to consider that previous studies in communication have sometimes required that the subject deal with the generated signal and sometimes with the intended message, and the experimental tasks may be quite disparate.

4. It is typically assumed that the talker and listener, in everyday situations, have about the same message sets. If an individual demonstrates that he is atypical in this respect, one ordinarily considers him socially imperceptive. In terms of the original schema, this may be the result of different perceptions in talker and listener of any of the five components or combinations of components.

Problems of this sort are not typically considered to be in the realm of appropriate study for the person interested in communication, though the model does indicate how they might be attacked experimentally.

5. Presence of the *Response Message* asserts that only if the listener alters his behavior as a result of the communication can communication be considered to have occurred. The response message need not be in the form of speech, though whatever form it may take, it can properly be considered equivalent to the generated signal of a communication in the other direction.

6. There is no necessary reason that a speech unit extracted from the received message need map isomorphically onto the generated signal. For example, we may note that the concept the linguist refers to as *phoneme* occurs as a perception; that is, it is a *Received Message*. There is a receiver operative in the communication prior to that point, and the receiver is an active element involving significant decision processes (see Figure 24). It would be expected that a change in decision behavior in the receiver leading to a different message would be preceded by a change in the signal, but there might well be large changes in the signal

leading to no change in the received message. Because of this, one must expect to find that a relatively invariant perception (received message) will show no single mapping—if, indeed. any at all—onto the generated signal, which may demonstrate high variability in repeated generations. Alternatively stated, there is no logical reason to assume that a percept, because it is unitary, need map invariantly onto any single signal dimension.

Because the message set is finite, one can detail its characteristics in the form of a propositional calculus, or finite state grammar,[4] which contains the message set available to the speaker in some communication gestalt. Change any factor of Figure 22 and you may alter the message set, but for each communication field there is some message set. All possible messages have some (theoretically) ascertainable Markov probability so that any element in a string may alter its expectation as one alters its environment, and the string may have its expectation altered by altering any of its constituent elements or their order. Each possible pathway (utterance) in the finite message set has some probability of occurrence, uniquely determined by all five elements considered in Figure 22. As previously noted, there is a general expectation that there will be much commonality in the message sets of the speaker and the receiver in a given situation. In many respects, the longer the communication the more constrained becomes the set of possible sentences from which any "next" sentence may be selected. By the same token, unless the speaker and receiver have some differences in their message sets so that the listener is continually being more or less surprised, the communication becomes progressively impoverished.[5]

The more constrained the communication, that is, the smaller the

[4] The reader interested in the operations involved in analyzing and evaluating a finite message set will find an explicit presentation in V. E. Giuliano, "Analog Networks for Word Association," *IEEE Transactions on Military Electronics*, 1963, MIL–7, 221–225. A more general discussion, perhaps of greater use to the general reader, is found in D. A. Norman, *Memory and Attention: An introduction to human information processing* (New York: Wiley, 1969), esp. Chap. 8, "Models of Memory," pp. 141–176.

[5] One samples for such commonality when chatting socially with relative strangers, and one relies heavily on the expectation of commonality in friends of long standing. It might be suggested that a new acquaintance who is instantly acceptable reveals himself as such in that he shows to a significant degree that he meets our expectations in areas of perception in which we have little tolerance for variation. Simultaneously, we are delighted if he also shows a significant lack of predictability ("full of surprises") in those areas (attitudes, knowledge and/or skill areas, or political opinions, for example) for which we have great tolerance for variation (see also Goffman, *The Presentation of Self in Everyday Life*).

set of messages from which the next message can be chosen, the less uncertainty the message can resolve (the less information it can transmit). Because this is a decision of the receiver, acting upon more or less complete information about all aspects of the situation (the components of Figure 22), one cannot adequately appraise a communication or measure intelligibility without consideration of the components of the receiver involved in such decision processes.[6]

We will consider an expansion of both the *Speaker* and *Receiver,* the latter being presented first:

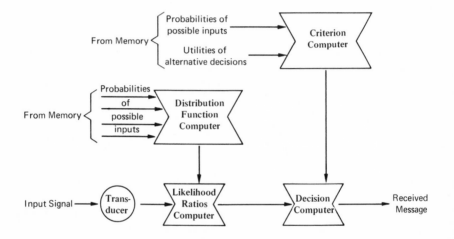

FIGURE 24. *The communication receiver (after Tanner)* .

The components of the model displayed as Figure 24 may not be as meaningful nor as psychologically real to the reader as previous schema, so that this level is presented in greater detail than previous levels have received.

The *Input Signal* to the *Receiver,* the *Generated Signal* as perturbed by the *Channel,* enters the *Transducer* which always changes the

[6] We pointed out earlier that articulation adequacy of an individual presents an interesting case in this respect. If a speaker produces an output with a phoneme substitution (that is, the generated signal is not congruent with the message as displayed on an instruction sheet), the receiver will probably "map" his received message onto the generated signal, whereas an output with a minor phoneme distortion will probably be mapped onto the intended message. As the distortion increases in severity, one may be evaluating the willingness of the listener to map onto the generated signal relative to his willingness to map onto the intended message, but one is not necessarily learning anything about the articulatory behavior of the speaker.

form of signal energy drastically but which also may, as in the case of a person with a hearing loss, impose its own peculiar perturbation upon the signal. The output of the *Transducer* is fed to a *Likelihood Ratio Computer* which determines the expectation (average mathematical probability) of the signal being one or another of a set of possible signals. This estimation is accomplished by calling upon memories about the characteristics of speech and nonspeech signals for comparison with the characteristic(s) of the input(s).

The process can be examined by considering the relatively simple task of establishing the basis for a decision that a particular signal arose from one or another distribution; that is, a discrimination. This discrimination involves the following stages:

1. Past observations made along the dimension X are drawn from memory in the form of distribution functions.

2. The signal observation (of some magnitude, Xo, along the dimension X) is now evaluated in terms of the retrieved distribution functions in order to derive an ordinate for the locus of the observation relative to distribution A and an ordinate for the observation relative to distribution B, as shown in Figure 25. Each distribution is divided

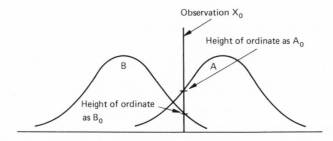

FIGURE 25. *Two-choice distributional discriminability and location of observation Xo expressed as a likelihood ratio.*

into two proportions by the ordinate. The proportions to the right of the ordinate, for distributions A and B (that is, the proportions of hits and false alarms, respectively) are determined by the location of the ordinate or, conversely, the location of the ordinate and the discriminability of the two distributions are derived from the hit and false alarm proportions. The ratio of the two proportions, called a likelihood ratio as it relates the likelihood that observation Xo arose from the distribution A relative to the likelihood that it arose from an alternative distribution B, uniquely characterizes Xo in terms of the stored memories about past observations labeled As and Bs.

3. The complex of material is delivered to a *Decision Computer,* which also receives an important set of information from a *Criterion Computer.*

4. The *Criterion Computer* calls upon stored information also, but of a somewhat different variety. These memories deliver estimates of the probability that one signal will be delivered relative to the probability that the other will (Does the first appear as frequently as the second? Ten times as frequently?) and in addition, supply estimates as to the cost to the receiver of making either decision—the signal was an *A;* the signal was a *B*—and the value to the receiver of making either decision.

5. This combination of signal probabilities and the utilities (values and costs) associated with each possible decision generates a criterion for use by the *Decision Computer.* The criterion is the collection of all points leading to the same decision. In this example, the criterion comprises all points with a likelihood ratio greater than the likelihood ratio of the criterion cutoff for the decision to be—the signal was an *A.* Observations of likelihood ratios less than that of the criterion cutoff make up the criterion resulting in the decision—the signal was a *B.*

6. The criteria are fed to the *Decision Computer,* which compares the signal observation (as a likelihood ratio) with the criteria (as ranges of likelihood ratios) and the output of the entire process is the decision—the message is ———, which appears as the *Received Message* in Figure 23.

It might be explained that the Receiver's Message Set supplies some portions of the knowledge necessary to the operation of the receiver. Exactly which portions of the knowledge are considered to come from it depends upon how one chooses, arbitrarily, to parcel the necessary processes and storage banks among Receiver, Message Set, and Message Ensemble.

Having arrived at the complex information-processing and decision-making tasks which are components of the receiver, so that one can explore the contribution of this portion of a communication system to the intelligibility of a message transmitted through the system, let us delineate the structure revealing the basic components involved in generating a spoken message by a speaker:

The still greater complexity of Figure 26 over that of Figure 25 indicates why this discussion of the speaker has followed that of the receiver.

The goal of the talker is to bring about some behavioral change in

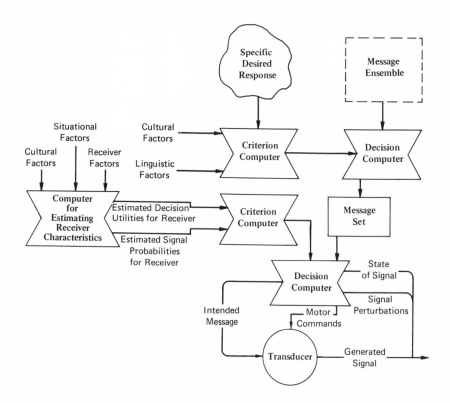

FIGURE 26. *The communication speaker.*

the listener. This behavioral reaction by the listener, taken within the totality of the situation schematized in Figure 22, can be any member of an enormous response repertoire, and so is schematized as an amorphous space labeled *Desired Response.* To bring about this desired response, the talker must energize the listener through the medium of a *Generated Signal,* having a high probability of effecting this behavior.

The schema asserts that the speaker calls upon a set of estimates of the characteristics of the receiver. These may be a set of memories of previous reactions of the receiver to various signal inputs in one situation or another. On the other hand, the particular target receiver may be a stranger to the speaker, who in this circumstance can only call upon various noncommunication characteristics of the receiver (or formalized modes of communication established by the culture) which, presumably, give insight into his expectable communication behavior (such as general appearance, posture, dress, and the like).

Ultimately, by some means, the talker must generate some estimates both of the receiver's expectations for certain signals and of the receiver's values and costs (the utilities) associated with these various signals with respect to the likelihood that a signal will motivate the desired response. These estimates of signal probabilities and associated utilities will be used to generate a criterion (or criteria) which will take from the infinite set *(Message Ensembles)* that small and finite set imputed to have some probability of generating the desired response and reducing this set (message set) to a single choice (intended message) having the highest probability of success in the task.[7]

The intended message is run through the motor speech system to form the spoken output. In the human being, this stage involves an active *Feedback* loop comparing the signal with the intended message, and introducing corrective motor commands when the isomorphism is disturbed.

This portion of the model, and indeed any portion, can be markedly expanded so that, for example, one can show a criterion computer-decision computer process handling the phonological component of the message, which is different from the computer's handling the choosing of the semantic message. Or one can introduce components dealing with the alteration of a CNS-stored message into a set of neural commands, to a set of muscle commands, to a set of articulator commands (into, through, and out of physiological "target range" locations), and so forth.

Many such expansions can be generated and can be illuminating for one or another purpose. Generally, however, we will not pursue any expansion. Rather we will use the speech communication model as a target of study so that we can uncover the kinds of data we require but do not yet have; we seek more comprehensive understanding of our simple model prior to expanding its complexity.

RESEARCH ON PERSONNEL

The model of the communication process immediately preceding points up the importance of the message set of the receiver in determining the content of any communication he will receive. Complete dis-

---

[7] I make no warrant that this process has two steps; it may have more or less. I desire to show that the speaker, in fact, can generate an infinite set of messages, only some finite set of which can be considered as having a probability greater than zero of motivating the desired response; and, inevitably, the speaker will deliver one of these.

belief in the possibility of a particular message (if such occurs in a human being) precludes receipt of that message. Therefore it is appropriate that we begin consideration of insights our model might provide for research by raising some questions about receivers and their a priori message sets.

A consideration not completely independent of our concern in Chapter 5 on what we teach pivots on the question of whether the clinical art is open to teaching. The two questions are partially independent because we may consider it appropriate to teach the same content whichever way we answer the latter question of the "teachableness" of the clinical art. However, there are implications for additional dimensions depending upon how we answer the latter question.

If we consider that the clinical art is *not* open to teaching, we must rapidly develop procedures to screen prospective entrants to the clinical field and subsequently devote our energies to sharpening the inherent skills of those who survive the initial screening. We show greater faith in our training procedures and in all of us previously trained and currently working at professional clinical careers if we adopt the alternative position that clinical arts can be taught and learned during a college-based training program. Therefore, we will adopt this latter stance and proceed to explore some questions about prospective changes in components of clinical training and their underlying research implications. First, however, we will fix upon a point that might be important for the alternative position that clinical art is not open to teaching and learning.

As a profession, we have virtually no data on the characteristics of an assisting therapist. And insofar as we do not know the necessary characteristics of a successful assisting therapist, it is difficult to assert that the characteristics can be taught. For example, there are several persons interested in detailing characteristics of successful psychotherapists. They adopt different approaches to research in the area and a variety of points of view. It is not germane that we consider particulars of all these various points of view because they would involve us in criteria of success, patient selection problems, considerations of clinical milieu in which therapy takes place, and a myriad of other considerations, none of which is specific to our problem; but we will consider one such.

One current point of view, an extension of the developments of interpersonal interaction promoted by Carl Rogers [8] is that of Charles

---

[8] C. R. Rogers, "The Therapeutic Relationship: Recent Theory and Research," *Australian Journal of Psychology*, 17 (1965), 95–108.

Truax,[9] who finds successful therapists achieve high ratings on three characteristics: genuineness, empathy, and nonpossessive warmth. As we said above, the general area of characteristics of assisting therapists is one about which psychologists find themselves in less than complete agreement and we are using a particular position for purposes of illustration only. Truax states that these three characteristics are not necessarily highly correlated, but any successful therapist requires two of the three. Of importance to us is Truax's finding that the three qualities can be taught only with great difficulty, if at all. Of these qualities, empathy seems altered most easily, but the clinical characteristics of genuineness and nonpossessive warmth seem resistant to long-lasting change.

So we can use the Truax formulations and results to point up the fundamental problem: if these or like characteristics are essential also to the successful speech and hearing therapist and if such personality dimensions cannot be taught, then training in speech and hearing should be given only to persons who pass some discriminating screening process, independently of any criteria of prior academic performance which may also be used as entrance criteria. However, we do not, on the average, employ such a screening technique early in student training, or prior to entrance to training. There is no a priori reason to believe the national examinations of The American Boards of Examiners in Speech Pathology and Audiology (ABESPA) are sensitive to such dimensions of necessary clinical characteristics, or even that objective examinations could be made sensitive to such dimensions were we able to say what the proper ones were. The entire issue is cloudy, deeply in need of research exploration and, perhaps of critical importance.

Let us return to the alternative and more comfortable position that components of clinical competence can be taught and learned, even though we cannot presently specify what these dimensions of competence comprise. Our chosen mode for this teaching/learning process should be some programmed procedure using the prototypical learning paradigm (response output, response evaluation, feedback, and success-contingent reward). We choose this mode because it explicates the structure used by the teacher. For example, if we use observation experiences as a systematic learning/teaching device and evaluate the growing competence of the observer, we have a systematic check on the perceptual categories being formed by observers.

What specific behaviors should we look at and how should we

---

[9] C. B. Truax, "The Empirical Emphasis in Psychotherapy: a Symposium. Effective Ingredients in Psychotherapy: An Approach to Unraveling the Patient-Therapist Interaction," *Journal of Consulting Psychology*, 10 (1963), 256-263.

quantify them? The previous discussion about what a potential therapist can or can not learn points out that, perhaps, we have too few data on what the appropriate perceptual categories should be. Presumably they will be better detailed with systematic study. In the interim, we will have the advantage of knowing what categories are being used, and can alter these as we gain insight into those categorization schemes that do seem to lead to clinical competence.

It is apparent that the criteria we have discussed carry with them social value judgments. In addition, the tasks performed in supervising and guiding patients and technicians (sub-professional personnel), many of whom will not share social class with their supervisors, involve the tells us that our value judgments reflect our social origins and strivings. To my knowledge, there has never been an investigation of the class clinician repeatedly in social judgments. There is much literature that structure of persons in speech and hearing. It seems that, particularly with the marked increase in therapeutic efficiency that behavioral engineering combined with programmed learning appears to afford, it becomes necessary for us to evaluate the influence of social background on criteria established in speech and hearing and transmitted by teachers in our college programs. Further, we must systematically insure that future generations of clinicians have knowledge of sociology sufficient to free them from such constraints in judgment as now may exist because of the origins of the members of the profession.

We need suggest only minimal additional discussion to the two areas of potential study discussed. The first of these is a study of socioeconomic origins and social views of speech and hearing clinicians as these things can be expected to influence the expectations of the clinician about others, and potentially to influence his judgments on the desirability or propriety of the speech or other characteristics of patients.

Further, the therapist will be attempting to manipulate the payoff matrix of the patient to insure motivating the patient to effect permanent change. Particularly is this true with the pediatric hearing-impaired, for whom the therapist must systematically supplement (or supply) a rational societal payoff underlying various decisions. If it is logical to assert that the therapist must consider and manipulate the patient's utility structure, then it is reasonable to ask if there are any systematic biases, on the average, in the utility structures of persons pursuing professional careers in speech and hearing.

These characteristics of a therapist, considered as a receiver in our model, may have significant impact or perhaps no impact on his decision processes. Our belief is that there appear to be no such class attitudes operative, though individual therapists may be guilty in this manner, but no data have appeared in the literature to support this or any alternative belief.

The second concern may be little more than a positive approach to many of the same characteristics. We must systematically and insightfully evaluate both our superior and our less-than-adequate clinicians, based on rating procedures perhaps not yet developed, to discover the attributes of assisting therapists. Subsequent to the completion of the task, we will face the even more difficult responsibility of developing techniques to assist our therapists-in-training to learn these assisting traits. But we must begin by discovering what they are.

If the clinician uses his own experiences and his perceptions of the reactions of others to various environmental situations to predict behavior of patients, then training of clinicians dealing with such predictions must accomplish two goals.

First of all, the pre-professional must be made aware of his own reactions, and thereby the expected reactions of patients, to kinds of speech and hearing problems wherein patients can be expected to have reactions like those of persons without such problems. Training must, secondly, sort out those speech problems for which the patient's reactions can be expected to differ from the reactions of the individual with normal speech so that the budding clinician can be trained in what these non-normal reactions are.

Probably the most obvious example of a person with a speech problem that alters his perceptions of his own speech as well as the speech of others is that of the stutterer. He seems to have atypical perceptions of the incidence of nonfluencies in speech so that he perceives "fluency" as a goal with a definition that is physiologically incapable of achievement.

Milisen, in the process of constructing theory about the occurrences of misarticulation in children, has gathered data that suggest that children are misperceptive of their own articulation as it is being produced.[10] He asserts that children make articulatory errors of which they are unaware though they have no difficulty identifying these same errors if the speech is stored and subsequently reproduced to the talker.

Additional examples can be cited for speech problems that seem to indicate aberrant perceptions of one's own speech. The author wishes to point up the advantages to the clinician of becoming aware of such conditions and, more importantly, of their implications.

[10] Milisen, "Articulatory Problems," *Speech Pathology.*

On the other side of the question, as to what kinds of speech or hearing disorders yield "normal" perceptions about one's own speech, we are in dire need of data. In the same way that a pimple on my face is infinitely large when I look at it in a mirror and yet perhaps completely unnoticed by anyone around me, there is some question as to whether anyone can come to therapy without a speech or hearing problem that has not been grossly magnified. We can only guess whether anyone can be expected to have an atypical (substandard) trait in our society, which seems to reward the young, healthy and beautiful, without the recognition of that trait bringing its own peculiar perceptual distortions.

Personal reaction systems often cause one to compensate for perceived defects. For example, some stutterers become abnormally fluent as a compensation for their perceived speech inadequacies, whereas others settle for a markedly taciturn, nonverbal existence. Demosthenes, the Greek orator who shouted over the roar of waves with a mouthful of pebbles, was presumed to have been a stutterer. In the same way, we discuss the "Napoleonic Complex" of atypically short men who strive for the acquisition of power. Let us not forget, however, that such persons do not necessarily have gross misperceptions about the importance of minor things to society in general. We are all too aware of the person who is successful on the basis of little more than an advantageous choice of parents, which made him somewhat taller than the average and gave him silver-tipped hair.

We might, as a first approximation, agree that one area of badly needed descriptive research is that of the subjective impression of those with speech and hearing problems about their own problems and their perceptions of "normal" and how deeply into their general attitudes they seem to generalize their own perceptions of being atypical. Sociologists of knowledge and attitude tell us that every man is the captive of his own view and the view of his subculture and his time.[11] We in speech and hearing have significant insights yet to be gathered about what kind of prisoner of his own speech defect a speech defective becomes. Whatever the dynamics of these perceptions might be, we must expose ourselves to them so that we might begin to appreciate the bases of behavior of our patients vis-à-vis their own speech and their behavior in the therapy situation.

For the moment, it appears that we might move away from both

---

[11] See, for example, K. Mannheim, *Ideology and Utopia* (New York: Harcourt, 1966).

perceptions and motivations of patients to consider behavior modification, at least for that group of patients willing to submit themselves to operant conditioning types of manipulations. We may note in passing that the proportion of all speech and hearing patients who are susceptible to such manipulation varies with the source one chooses to quote. However, such individuals do demonstrate that their behavior and seemingly their attitudes about their own speech are both open to manipulation and remediation. There is little doubt that for the class of patient who will perform such programmed tasks, the expectation of success, given a well-designed program, approaches a certainty.

Should we consider it strange that a child will markedly alter his speech behavior in some permanent way for a bit of candy, and that an adult will make the same or even a much more difficult change, in the sense that he has that much more practice to overcome, for an occasional smile?

Without getting involved in a full discussion of the power of a smile, the rewards for which men strive, or other characteristics involved in payoff matrices appropriate to performance of people of one kind or another, the point is evident that we have sizable insights into how to increase, maintain, or reduce motivations in ourselves and in others. We do not require instruction in ways to manipulate such human traits so much as we require conscious consideration and structuring of what we already know, plus some insightful research into patients' perceptions of their own speech and hearing problems. We realize that behavior is open to simple and varied reinforcers of both a positive and negative variety, and that such reinforcers can have a profound effect upon the patient's behavior. However, the fact that we think we know how to deal with the patient, even though he may have aberrant perceptions of his own speech, should not keep us from an all-out evaluation of his self-perceptions, and some reasonable appraisal of the importance of these must precede the formulation of any major advance in therapy with the speech- or hearing-impaired.

RESEARCH ON SPEECH CHARACTERISTICS

The implications of the model have been most strongly represented by examples in the area of therapy. Many of these illustrative examples, in turn, imply knowledge not currently available to the profession, thereby giving rise to a series of parameter-estimating tasks. Our goals in estimating parameters are to provide the normative data against which background we can evaluate findings on any single patient. The parameters we typically will have interest in evaluating are shape, variance and distinctiveness of distributions. We need such information on a variety of voice qualities, a variety of "normal" fluency rates, and a variety of normal prosodic patterns. In the next section (research on attitudes) we will look at many of these same things from the point of view of obtaining the perceptions of persons with some communication problem. Both this section and the next deal with normal speech traits; in this section the focus is on normal perceptions of the variables and in the next section the focus is on potential differences between normal perceptions and impaired perceptions of communication.

The accomplishment of these estimation tasks will allow us to determine the shapes and variances of the distributions under consideration, as well as their distinctiveness. Given this information, we can construct simple tasks to reveal the criteria of a clinician, a clinician-in-training, a patient, that same patient sometime later in therapy, matched samples of patients under different therapeutic procedures, matched samples of patients under different schedules of therapy, and comparable issues.

The quantification that becomes available because of this application of the model need be no more complex than a percentage-correct measure or some other performance index (and two such measures are presented in a later section) for such a test as, for example, discrimination of a difference in phonemes, or a difference in linguistically distinctive features, or a difference in voice qualities. If one can presume the availability of some instrumentation, then performance might be measured for correct production of non-nasal vowels; or for the ability to view a film associated with a case history and arrive at an appropriate education recommendation, or an appropriate therapy beginning, among others.

For many of these training procedures, what is required is the construction of a scaled series of signals (such as nasal voice quality) and determination of an accepted expert criterion. The student showing comparable skill at classification demonstrates his achievement of competence in the matter under test. Perhaps equally important, the quantification realized in constructing the scale brings greater semblance of order to our general understanding of the skills necessary to the clinician.

Another point of interest raised by these considerations is the possibility of optimizing the strategy for teaching the knowledge associated with the acquisition of clinical skills. What should be the appropriate mixture of material, i.e., observation plus practice plus classroom lecturing plus coffee-break interaction? What should be the content of the third year of a five-year program or, more generally, what particular aspects should come at each academic level? Where should one begin a new graduate student, new to the discipline, whose professed interest is the research process in speech and hearing?

By implication, any variable on which we are likely to need to know the location of criteria of master clinicians, patients, teachers, or other subpopulations of interest represent variables open to experimental study. Many such variables are referred to and discussed in succeeding sections.

RESEARCH ON ATTITUDES

A great portion of the suggested research is based in the idea that the model is one that has perceptions of the world as an explicit base, and we have all too few insights into people's perceptions of events as complex and transitory as speech, particularly if the people in question have problems in the media of communication.

One area for research would include perceptions of various voice qualities by normal persons, particularly with reference to the perceiver's judgment of "normal" voice quality and the relationship between the perceived deviation from normal and the attractiveness of the voice quality, per se. Is there a correlation between voice quality as perceived, and estimated physical or psychological well-being? Is there a correlation between perceived voice quality and estimated intelligence? estimated leadership potential? estimated socio-economic status? A second area of research would explore the correlations of speaking rates and these perceptions of psychosocial ratings. Still a third area might pursue articulatory precision and dialect-revealing pronunciations and their correlations with psychosocial perceptions. All three of these lines of research are concerned with giving us some appreciation of the importance of more or less "goodness" in defining attitudes of listeners toward speakers.

A corollary concern for each of these approaches is a determination of what persons with varying magnitudes of speech or hearing disorders of each type consider to be the characteristic attitudes of other people to them. Are there aberrations in perception routinely to be found in speech defectives and, if so, how aberrant and destructive might they be?

Still another area of research, impinging upon consideration in the decisions about the age at which therapy should begin for public school children with functional articulation disorders, is that of estimating the perceptions of individuals (in particular, but not restricted to, school teachers) about children with such misarticulations. If the disorder does not entail a significant social cost to the child, we might be more willing to revise our consideration about the time for beginning therapy with these children when we face the recurring problem of choosing among too many patients.

The entire set of studies arises from that portion of the model suggesting that the perceptions of a large number of people for any quality that can be thought of as complex in nature and representing a synthesis of a large number of independent factors, each of which is as likely to influence the final judgment in one direction as in the other, would distribute themselves normally on the decision axis. The aim of the studies would be to allow one to evaluate the mean and variance of each distribution obtained from the perceptions of normal talkers and those obtained from defective talkers. In this way we can begin to deal with the significance of any speech-defective's perceptions about the relationship, in the mind of his listener, between his speech defect and aspects of his personality. Are there yet-to-be-discovered characteristic relationships for listeners and, if so, is the speech defective insightful about them?

RESEARCH ON THERAPY AND EVALUATION

Probably one of our most urgent needs is for additional insights into what behavioral traits of clinicians facilitate therapy. What kinds of feedback facilitate behavioral change of lasting value in the various dimensions of speech? Can repeated success in a clinical task be considered an intrinsic value growing to some asymptotic level? Might it instead properly be considered to have some heavy merit early in therapy but be less motivating in later therapy? What kinds of feedback enhance the value of success? How rigorous or stringent a criterion of success should be adopted, and should the criterion alter during therapy? If so, toward greater or lesser stringency?

Perhaps we can make these questions somewhat more operational by considering an exemplary case. Let us suppose that we have two hearing-handicapped patients of approximately equal capacities, however such capacities might be measured. Both obtain a significant portion of their communication input by speech-reading. One of these persons uses a lax criterion in reading others, while the other uses a much stricter criterion. In other words, speech reader 1 guesses frequently about the topic under discussion, about what a particular talker probably said, and the like, and he is frequently incorrect. Speech reader 2 guesses much less frequently and therefore makes fewer errors. He also understands fewer conversations.

In terms of our previous paragraph, which is the tactic to be recommended? Is the lower success proportion of patient 2 (of all the conversations that he could participate in, he participates successfully in fewer than does patient 1) in some sense better than that of patient 1, the latter understanding but also misunderstanding more conversations? Patient 2 certainly has fewer failures than patient 1, but most of the time he is out of the conversation whereas patient 1 is in the conversation more but frequently on the wrong track. Earlier, in the chapter on therapy, we asserted that increasing the output of a patient in therapy was a goal for therapy and should therefore be rewarded. Is the appropriate analogue in the present example that of increasing the guesses of the patient, thereby increasing both the hit rate and the false alarm rate, in which case patient 1 is the more successful? Or should we maintain that the patient achieve success most frequently when he participates, in which case patient 2, showing fewer errors, should be considered as having a better strategy?

Hopefully, the example reinforces our felt need for serious thought about what therapy is to do and how it is to do it, accompanied by some empirical studies to help us along with our thinking. Our particular example posed questions about facilitating behavioral traits of patients. Before we return to comparable considerations of facilitating behavioral traits of clinicians, let us consider some additional ideas.

We are all at least vaguely aware that certain types of postural attitudes in a listener will cause a talker to increase his loudness and precision of articulation. Is it good therapy to train a hearing-handicapped individual to use these postural poses to influence his communication milieu? If so, what particular postures should he learn and what magnitude of advantage can we expect him to achieve?

What kinds of therapy would be effective, and with what relative efficiencies, in teaching the hearing-handicapped to deal with those properties of signals that he does receive, in order to optimize his probability for correctly recognizing the message? Experiments directed toward rationalizing this latter goal might properly employ a kind of reductionist approach. That is, one can evaluate the gain in obtained intelligence for a set of messages coming about from training the subject to attend to a count of the number of syllables, to attend to the tense of a sentence, and to identify the sentence as being one of a set using a particular prosodic pattern (emphatic statement, question, and so forth).

RESEARCH ON AUDIOLOGICAL EVALUATION

The question of what behaviors of clinicians facilitate goal achievement is a particularly fascinating one, particularly in audiology and most particularly in the evaluative process. What does it mean to undertake an audiological assessment of the hearing of an uncooperative patient? We have already noted the profound difference between sensitivity to signals and hearing of signals. While both measures are influenced by the expectations and motivations of the patient so that both might be markedly altered in magnitude of any measure by the behavior of the clinician, the former tends to be some criterion measure on "hearing"/"nonhearing" of a signal, whereas the latter involves complex decision processing with perhaps associated matching of neural patterns and the like.

In order to give proper consideration to the question of evaluating the hearing of an uncooperative patient we must step back and examine some larger questions of audiological evaluation.

The field of audiology has stressed these two types of diagnostic measure during its post-World War II history. Two examples of the first type, an estimate of the patient's sensitivity to signals of various kinds, are: pure tone of continuous or interrupted delivery, and the difference limen. The second type of diagnostic measure has been some index of the utility of the information the patient does receive. An example of this latter type of measure would be a speech intelligibility score.[12]

The patient's active contribution of decision processes to the result obtained on the second type of test has never been in dispute, though it may not yet be fully understood. Egan discussed the necessity of acquainting the subject with the speech materials to be used when he first developed the lists that served and continue to serve as a source for

[12] The term intelligence is introduced here because we need a term in addition to intelligibility. For example, when the performance on a speech test is measured in percentage-correct, a subject willing to guess about an uncertain transmission will score higher than a subject who refuses to respond, even though they have comparable auditory functioning. Therefore, we will use the term *intelligence* to mean the score obtained by a subject when that score reflects both signal discriminability and subject response strategy, and we will reserve *intelligibility* to mean a measure of signal discriminability when the response strategy is one appropriate to maximizing performance.

much clinical testing.[13] Goldiamond and Hawkins should have removed any residual doubt in the mind of anyone as to what could happen if the clinician ignores the subject's decision processing. [14]

The contributions of the patient's expectations—his decision processing—in the sensitivity measure has also been appreciated in some ways by most clinicians but not as pervasively as one might hope. For example, there is a very general agreement that a patient's ascending threshold is less sensitive than his descending threshold. But if one stops to consider the theoretical basis of a threshold as being that level of input below which the signal is *never* perceived and above which the signal is *always* perceived, how can that level be influenced by preceding signal levels? To put that another way, if the last signal input level influences perception of the signal, there must be more than one threshold, or, more properly, an infinitude of thresholds.

Again, if I instruct a patient to signal when he hears a "tone" and, on retest, instruct him to signal when he hears any "sound," I can record more than one threshold. If I deliver a shock when he does not respond to a signal but no shock when he responds in the absence of a signal, I can improve his threshold (increase his sensitivity?). Indeed, anything I do to alter his willingness to guess about the presentation of a signal will alter his threshold; anything I do to alter the value or cost of saying, Yes, there is a signal! when no signal is presented, will alter his threshold. Isn't one then forced to conclude, along with Swets, that there is no threshold at all or, more exactly, an infinitude of thresholds? [15] In terms of our model, what we call a threshold is nothing more than a criterion

[13] J. P. Egan, "Articulation Testing Methods," *The Laryngoscope*, 58 (1948), 955–991.

[14] I. Goldiamond and W. F. Hawkins, "Vexierversuch: the Log Relationship between Word-Frequency and Recognition Obtained in the Absence of Stimulus Words," *Journal of Experimental Psychology*, 56 (1958), 456–463. Goldiamond and Hawkins trained a panel of subjects to respond in a forced-choice write-down task to a series of words presented tachistoscopically. The subjects were trained to expect individual words with varying frequencies of occurrence and were continued in training until they demonstrated that they had internalized the experimenal word-frequency bias. They were then put into an experimental situation and, following each of a set of tachistoscopic flashes, had to write down the word presented. Subjects responded with the words used in training, as they were restricted to the use of only this set, and did so with the word frequencies used during their training. However, there were no signals used in the second part of the experiment—the light flashes projected no words at all.

   If, as in the above experiment, the subject displays his expectations about the signal when he is led to believe there will be a signal, one must conclude that his response behavior will reflect and be influenced by the same kinds of expectations about signals in the audiological evaluation situation.

[15] J. A. Swets, "Is There a Sensory Threshold?," *Science*, 134 (1961), 168–177.

cutoff and is open to the influence of signal probabilities, the probability a signal will exceed some arbitrary loudness, and in addition, the values and costs of saying, Yes, I heard a tone.

In spite of this kind of logical onslaught, if audiologists continue to make the assumption that some kind of estimate of tonal acuity *must* be derived clinically, is there any assistance we can offer? As a preliminary to answering this question in the affirmative, let us explore some of the dimensions of tonal audiometry.

Our discussion starts with an appreciation that modern-day psychophysics, intellectually and in its instrumentation, has revealed three types of inadequacies in current tonal-signal procedures:

1. The primary inadequacy with audiometric procedures is the concept of a threshold. We have just dealt with some of the inadequacies of this concept and we should now appreciate how little the clinician subscribes to this notion in his day-by-day clinical dealings. We are all familiar with the influence on our results of fatigability, instructions to the patient, clinical conduct of the examiner, and so forth. And yet every evaluation yields a threshold curve which, while not the sole determiner of any clinical judgment, is a weighty factor in determining the procedures and recommendations of the examiner.

2. A second error that the examiner makes is that the patient is not given freedom to sort his decisions into two categories. He can answer Yes, but he does not routinely have the option of answering No. Such a constraint may or may not operate to the disadvantage of the patient, but it certainly operates to the disadvantage of the clinician. This might best be discussed by pointing out that the clinician should be able to separate patient responses into four categories, as displayed in the 2 × 2 matrix following:

	PATIENT REPORT	
	Signal Present	No Signal Present
signal delivered	1	3
no signal delivered	2	4

I have labeled the boxes 1–4 for purposes of facilitating discussion. Note that boxes 1 and 3 are the responses to which you typically attend, the former directly and the latter by imputation. Very occasionally a patient will respond with a #2 response (indicating he heard a tone when none was presented) but the clinician routinely ignores such "false positives." Also note that attending only to type 1 and 3 responses restricts the clinician to evaluating a confounded response situation, without any means to sort between the contribution of the patient's sensitivity and the patient's willingness to reach the decision "I will say 'Yes'." If one obtained types 2 and 4 decisions, in addition to the 1 and 3 decisions, he would have additional estimates of the patient's willingness to reach a decision and could remove this factor from the results in boxes 1 and 3, leaving a less contaminated measure of sensitivity.

3. A third complicating and incorrect assumption is that the clinician and the patient share common observation intervals. The clinician appears to operate as though the patient begins to listen only when he, the examiner, depresses the signal key to deliver a tonal signal. The examiner releases the key after a short presentation interval and, if the patient has not said Yes during the presentation interval, credits him with a response of No—or the equivalent state of having sensitivity poorer than that of the signal presentation level.

In fact, the patient has been in a continuous observation interval since his last positive response and, if low signal levels have recently been in use, may have begun to wander in attention or may have begun to concentrate more on listening because of his mounting anxiety about the lack of inputs. Either result comes about over time (as the voluminous literature on vigilance will attest) and both results indicate a varying criterion in the patient that may be interpreted as a variation in sensitivity. One might point out, parenthetically, that it is correctly interpreted as a variation in sensitivity of the individual, if that is what one presumes to measure in the clinical situation, but it should not be mistaken as a variation in sensitivity of the end organ, which is the assumed basis for such measurement. However one cares to characterize the situation, the examiner turns his attention on and off with the signal presentation key, but the patient does not.

Now that all three misconceptions complicating audiometric pure-tone results have been delineated, let me return for a minute to the threshold concept. The measure used to derive the threshold confounds two aspects, both of which are important to the patient and therefore to the examiner.

Ramsdell presented an insightful view of some of the psychological concomitants of hearing loss and the almost two decades since have reinforced the generality and depth of his observations.[16] The hearing handicapped individual, many times, alters in personality as his loss continues. To the extent that such personality constriction occurs, which alters the willingness of that patient to say Yes under routine "threshold" evaluative procedures, one would achieve results interpreted as a reduc-

---

[16] D. A. Ramsdell, "The Psychology of the Hard-of-Hearing and the Deafened Adult." in Davis and Silverman, *Hearing and Deafness*, third ed.

tion in sensitivity though they may reflect no change in end-organ functioning. The clinical evaluation would be incorrect and the therapy misguided and, in all likelihood, ineffectual.

What the clinician should obtain, if he can, is a sensitive measure of the stability of the subject's decision behavior about auditory signals as well as a measure of his sensitivity (magnitude of loss) to auditory signals. Both these measures are in the threshold as measured and should be sorted out so that both might be utilized.

At this time, Békésy audiometry cannot be said to remove any of the problems involved in the confounding of these two measures. Automatic audiometry may add only additional information about the patient's willingness to reach a decision, insofar as he must now decide both that he hears it and that he no longer hears it, without giving us any leverage toward distinguishing that type of his decision behavior or the type of decision behavior necessary to effective therapy planning and management. If the measured "threshold" of the Békésy audiogram can be shown to relate to an uncontaminated estimate of the patient's sensitivity, and if some aspect of the Békésy "swing" can be shown to relate to the estimate of decision behavior that effective therapy planning requires, then the Békésy procedure could serve in a continuing function. It seems that, at this time, there is little ground for making either assertion for results of such automatic audiometry, though Shepherd and Goldstein,[17] and others,[18] have displayed some interesting beginnings.

We could go on to discuss a number of alternative approaches, variously objective, which can be used to discern when we have a patient who is set upon misleading us as to his acuity. But knowing that his acuity is no worse than some value doesn't tell us how much better it might be and gives us no genuine insight into his ability to use what auditory signals he does receive. Unfortunately, as long as our society rewards illness (as in the Veterans Administration paying compensation for hearing loss and increased compensation for increased loss) it will be advantageous to the patient's pocketbook for him to appear more ill

[17] D. C. Shepherd and R. Goldstein, "Relation of Békésy Tracings to Personality and Electrophysiologic Measures," *Journal of Speech and Hearing Research*, 9 (1966), 385–411, and "Intrasubject Variability in Amplitude of Békésy Tracings and its Relation to Measures of Personality," *Journal of Speech and Hearing Research*, 11 (1968), 525–535.

[18] C. F. Greenspan and K. C. Pollack, "Response Variability and Personality Factors in Automated Audiometry," *Journal of Auditory Research*, 9 (1969), 386–390.

than he is and not to cooperate in an examination designed to minimize his otopathological insult.

Considered in a slightly more abstract manner, we desire an estimate of the hearing competence of the patient, but are restricted to some aspect of his performance. So long as the audiologist considers himself as a manipulator of equipment, which insures his objectivity, he will not even be aware that the possibility exists for his behaviors to be influential in the measures he derives from his patients, and will not consider the topic a fit subject for research. But we must systematically evaluate the interaction of clinician's behaviors and patient's behaviors or, as perhaps the only reasonable alternative, refer to another professional person (psychiatrist, psychologist, social worker) any patient who appears less than optimally cooperative.

RESEARCH ON AUDIOLOGICAL THERAPIES

When we move away from the needed research on sensitivity or acuity in hearing to take up the more significant question of maximizing the yield of therapy (that is, dealing with the decision processes of the patient and helping him to optimize them), we probably do best to concentrate upon the patient during and after the sessions in which his hearing aid is fitted. The conditions we can be assumed to have met in this case are that any medical/surgical assistance that can be offered the patient has already transpired and we have, more or less successfully, determined the maximum to be expected from electro-acoustic assistance to the patient. Our motivation in viewing the problem in this manner is to deal both with needed research on hearing aids and needed research on hearing therapy.

The first question we can ask grows out of the clinical insight that a hearing-handicapped patient likes the sound quality with which he is familiar even though it may not yield the greatest recognition test score (intelligence). We may presume, correctly or not, that his degree of satisfaction with quality will interact with his motivation in a testing situation so that he will do less well with progressively deviating sound qualities. (The fact that individual patients may not do so under clinical hearing aid testing suggests that there may be even larger differences in the potential assisting abilities of aids than we believe even now.) The implication is that the results we obtain in a hearing-aid fitting may be partially determined by the patient's reactions to the frequency response and distortion characteristics of the instruments under test. As a research problem, it may well be the case that the best predictor of a patient's scores with different hearing aids is his rating of satisfaction with their sound qualities.[19] However, if one were to do such research, he should probably use talkers of both sexes and contextual materials in the listening tasks on which the patient would base his semantic differential ratings.

A second implication is that the patient's intelligence score with an instrument should increase as he becomes more familiar with it, regardless of the intelligence he receives on first evaluation. If this is true, can we derive some means of being able to predict the final intelligence score so that we can evaluate therapy progress and have a reasonable goal for estimating appropriate termination?

Further, if we can derive a measure for repeated use to obtain the shape of the function of changing intelligence, then we will have a means of evaluating the efficiencies of different therapeutic approaches. Also we will have the beginnings for evaluating the quality of the fit. As long as a patient may unknowingly work harder during an evaluation of a hearing aid whose sound characteristics he likes than he does for one that seems less satisfactory, and as long as we cannot estimate how well he should be able to function after fitting, familiarization, and therapy, we cannot legitimately be satisfied that we have done all that is appropriate to our professional obligation.

An additional associated domain of study is the relative validity of starting a hearing-aid familiarization process with the "response" giving the patient the maximum (for that date) obtained intelligence and using therapeutic procedures to assure that he will wear the hearing-aid long enough to accustom himself to it, as opposed to fitting him with a hearing-aid that sounds familiar and comfortable and gradually altering its response to achieve the maximal intelligence setting.

Even at this time there must be a wealth of data in the files of individual hearing-aid dealers that could give us some insights into these very problems if we could get our colleagues in the hearing-aid business to compile and evaluate such data. What proportion of dealers in any given year fit patients with fitting A of instrument X and why did they think the fitting was better than fitting B, or of fitting A of instrument Y?

Two needs underlying these kinds of evaluation strategies are immediately apparent. One is for a set of contextual materials that will be sensitive to differences in communication systems, including both the patient and the hearing aid. The other need is for a surveying technique

[19] S. Zerlin, "A New Approach to Hearing-Aid Selection," *Journal of Speech and Hearing Research,* 5 (1962), 370–376.

and instrument that can be used to index the magnitude of difficulty an individual experiences in his activities of daily living. The early work in this direction was that of Davis and his co-workers in their efforts to develop a Social Adequacy Index (SAI) for hearing.[20] Perhaps an approach that will separate acuity problems and decision (personality approach) problems will increase the effectiveness of the measures and move us closer to success.

We raised the question in Chapter 3 of the importance of binaural hearing to the person whose hearing is impaired. Hopefully, part of the descriptive information we would obtain from a new SAI would concern the differences experienced by patients with more or less hearing and more or less binaurally matched hearing. There is a voluminous literature concerning primarily binaural hearing of tonal signals in noise that deals with the advantage of binaural hearing.[21] This literature is restricted to well-trained subjects who hear normally and, for reasons expressed both earlier in the work and in a later section of this chapter (having to do with different expectations in signal reception by normally hearing and hearing-impaired listeners), cannot reasonably be used to predict the performances of hearing-impaired subjects for speech signals. Few studies have been undertaken that deal with binaural hearing applications to the impaired, but the interested reader can find some beginning in the bibliography.[22]

RESEARCH ON TRAINING

So much of Chapter 5 asserts the need for a different perspective, a reevaluation of our current methods, that a reader might be led to the conclusion that the product of our present training programs is much less adequately trained than he could be or should be. We do not know whether this is true. Further, while we can derive needed research areas and topics by considering teaching and learning within the framework of our model, we would in most cases be duplicating efforts taking place

[20] Davis, "The Articulation Area and the Social Adequacy Index for Hearing," *The Laryngoscope*, 58, 761–778, and "Information theory: Three Applications of Information Theory to Research in Hearing," *Journal of Speech and Hearing Disorders*, 17 (1952), 189–197.

[21] Much of this literature appears in the *Journal of the Acoustical Society of America* and deals with the differences required in the level of the masker, the Masking Level Difference (MLD), to yield equivalent performance under monaural listening or differing binaural hearing conditions.

[22] For a presentation of some of the clinical issues and problems, see Heffler and Schultz, "Some Implications of Binaural Signal Selection for Hearing-Aid Evaluation."

in many schools and colleges of education around the country. The problems of how to accomplish professional training in a college of arts and sciences or in a university graduate school are not problems unique to speech and hearing but, again, are under consideration in multiple locations throughout our college and university population.

Therefore, we will detail little in the way of research in this section and restrict ourselves to three areas that are pressing and important. The first of these is some systematic study of the breadth of observation necessary to give a young undergraduate the sufficient experience preceding his introduction to first-person clinical interaction. How much observation does he need, of what types and in what mixture, and how do we evaluate the yield from his exposure so that we can come to some justifiable decisions?

The second area of needed research, equally difficult, is that which will reveal for us what the supervisory skills are that contribute to the learning and maturation processes of the clinician. Are superior supervisors, like superior clinicians, born with the gift or can they learn it? And, even more important, what is it? If we build a scale (or scales) rating clinicians, can we also build scales rating supervisors so we can begin to see what common features they all display or from what larger set of common features they all seem to sample?

A final and more researchable area of needed work is that of building scales of representative speech disorders which can be used to achieve some uniformity in placement of criterion cuts from training program to training program and from clinician to clinician. We indicated earlier our support of the work on such scales that has been pursued by Sherman and her students for almost two decades.[23] Her endeavors have enjoyed little professional acceptance but we must move toward some consistency, and the Sherman approach offers the needed validity, ease of distribution, and so forth.

RESEARCH ON SPEECH AND HEARING PHENOMENA

The central concern in speech therapy is articulation. The elementary school clinician spends approximately 70 percent of his time dealing with articulatory precision. Much of the therapy in pathological areas (cleft palate, cerebral palsy, hearing loss) is directed toward in-

---

[23] See Sherman, "Clinical and Experimental Use of the Iowa Scale of Severity of Stuttering," *Journal of Speech and Hearing Disorders*, 17, 316–320. Also Sherman and Moodie, "Four Psychological Scaling Methods Applied to Articulation Defectiveness," *Journal of Speech and Hearing Disorders*, 20, 352–358.

creasing articulatory precision also. We suggested in Chapter 4 that there should be systematic exploration of three questions relating the patient's articulation to our ability to understand him; that is, the relationship between the severity of a misarticulation and the intelligibility of a patient, the relationship between the attractiveness of a misarticulation and the intelligibility of a patient, and the relationship between the persistence of a misarticulation and the intelligibility of a patient. None of these questions is of overwhelming importance, but all deal with our area of greatest expenditure of energy as therapists and we would do well to learn more about the perceptual dynamics of listeners for misarticulations in talkers.

Fairbanks, in his very insightful work, differentiated two types of feedback: feedback for control and feedback for estimation.[24] It might be fruitful to consider that memory-stored motor-production distributions arise from a control function, whereas perception distributions arise from an estimation function. In the first case, one is asking if the production, as viewed by way of motor feedback, is representative of the (ideal) target output (or is within appropriate criterial limits) that the talker desires to produce. In the second case, one is asking in what criterion, or what range, the input falls so that some decision can be made about its linguistic identification. That is to say, in the first case one begins with a class and accepts or rejects an utterance as being within the class. If the utterance is accepted, the talker continues; if not, he repeats, rephrases, and so forth. In the second case, feedback for estimation, one starts with the utterance and tries to pin a label on it in order to continue to understand the incoming message.

To use a very simple analogy, in the feedback for control one has a lock and acts to insure that a given key, as produced, fits it; in feedback for estimation, one has a key and tries to find the lock it opens.

The individual with acceptable articulation engages in both tasks as he produces speech. He monitors his own output for control and also, typically, serves as his own listener. But Milisen's data on the inability of children to recognize their own errors in production and the ability to recognize these same errors when tape-reproduced, would suggest that the two tasks are not of equivalent importance when conducted simultaneously, because the control judgment overrides the estimation judgment if they are in disagreement.[25] These same data, in the light of this hypothesized explanation, lead to the conclusion that training in auditory discrimination should not, by itself, alleviate the misarticulation problem. So let us look at it from another angle.

[24] G. Fairbanks, *Experimental Phonetics: Selected Articles.*
[25] Milisen, "Articulatory Problems," *Speech Pathology.*

We have tried throughout this presentation to maintain a necessary distinction between the terms "signal" and "stimulus." It might be good for us to examine the differences between the terms again at this time as a means of focusing on the causes of the problem of functional articulation difficulty.

We have considered, and implicitly defined, the concept of a signal many times—the signal comprises the characteristics of the energy that impinge upon the sensory end organs. The stimulus is defined as the portions of the signal to which the individual attends and it must be considered as sharply different from the signal in the same way that perceptibility differs from perception. It differs because the signal, in becoming a stimulus, has had its properties altered by the sensory receptors, which introduce their own properties onto any signal, and by the weighting given to the received properties by the person processing the transduced signal. In terms that we have used previously, the stimulus can be considered as the signal properties, transmitted through the end organ, and squeezed onto a decision axis; the latter involving paying more or less (great to zero) attention to various aspects of the message. We can say that the concept of a stimulus involves first, a signal and second a decision process on some (weighted) aspects of the signal.

With respect to evaluating functional articulatory problems, one can ask two questions about perception without ever considering production. The first is: Does the subject child use the same stimulus as the normal child? or: Does he attend to the same properties of the signal? The second question is: Does he use the same criterion cutoff?

If one or both the questions can be shown to strike upon a source of difficulty for the child in the sense that his behavior differs from that of the normal child, then the model will have demonstrated its utility in structuring the problem and will also reveal the appropriate structure for remedying the problem.

A more difficult area for research, but one of much greater significance to the individual patient, is that of speech-reading. The patient deriving a significant portion of his speech communication through his visual system places an overwhelming burden on a system already overworked by acting as a substitute for the auditory system for nonspeech signals. Further, speech communication is not designed to have distinctive visual elements as is a semaphore system, for example, so that understanding speech by reading only or primarily its visual components is at best an exceedingly difficult task. It seems that one could pursue a fruitful line of research into the components of speech-reading that would deal with the entire process by evaluating its components to find their relative abilities to reduce the receiver's uncertainty about the message. For example, a synthetic speech-reading orientation that seeks to identify the topic early in the processing of the input is using such an information-theory approach better than an analytic orientation focusing on the sequential identification of words or syllables.

Linguists and others interested in problems of a linguistic nature, particularly those pursuing applications of the transformational model of the structure of grammar, have concerned themselves with two levels of linguistic production or linguistic comprehension, the two levels being designated as *performance* and *competence*.

Chomsky discusses the terms and delineates their relationship in the following short pasage:

> Linguistic theory is concerned primarily with an ideal speaker-listener, in a completely homogeneous speech-community, who knows its language perfectly and is unaffected by such grammatically irrelevant conditions as memory limitations, distractions, shifts of attention and interest, and errors (random or characteristic) in applying his knowledge of the language in actual performance . . . To study actual linguistic performance, we must consider the interaction of a variety of factors, of which the underlying competence of the speaker-hearer is only one . . . We thus make a fundamental distinction between *competence* (the speaker-hearer's knowledge of his language) and *performance* (the actual use of language in concrete situations). Only under the idealization set forth in the preceding paragraph is performance a direct reflection of competence.[26]

Our present interest in considering the dichotomy is that it may illuminate some of the ground common to those in speech and hearing and those in linguistics, and it may assist the reader in understanding some of the motivations for the research proposed in this chapter. From the viewpoint of our central concern, one can interpret the performance-competence dichotomy in several ways. For example, we could assert that one's performance—some present measure—could be used to derive an efficiency-type measure by comparison with his competence—his best performance after training. The basis of this argument is that the difference between the two is definitional, strictly a matter of how one wished to employ his cutoff insofar as performance is the behavior routinely observed because it is high-probability behavior. Competence is low-probability behavior in that it will be displayed only on those few occasions when circumstances require the unusual response. One does not typically display the limits of his performance—his competence—so that it must be systematically elicited by experiment. The subject's attention is drawn to his own performance in such circumstances because

---

[26] N. Chomsky, *Aspects of the Theory of Syntax* (Cambridge: MIT Press, 1965), pp. 3–4.

the payoff for maximizing performance is high, and he (the subject) will improve in performance if he can. Experimentally, we should expect a varying estimate until he reaches a plateau that represents his true maximum (competence) for the experimental situation in which he finds himself.

This line of argument grows out of an economy-of-effort hypothesis. Those things a person must do routinely and repeatedly, he does easily and can accomplish in a variety of ways because he has many experiences in doing so, even though one particular way may be most efficient. Any single, though perhaps repeated, measure of his performance will display only some portion of his repertoire. But if one elicits behavior of a low probability, the subject will have had little earlier experience with it and will not previously have had much opportunity to vary his approaches to that same act. With repeated experience, he will vary his approach as he seeks to optimize his performance. If we evaluate performance, we will derive a varying measure until the subject stabilizes at the limit he can achieve in the sense that his performance would not be expected to improve with additional practice. I would only caution that additional practice, with the processing of signals as complex as speech, must be defined in the realm of thousands of trials of practice, not fifty or even several hundred.[27]

[27] There are few data speaking directly to this issue, except perhaps in the area of second language learning, although I have been unable to locate an appropriate illustration in that literature. A paper by W. P. Tanner, Jr., *Statistical Decision Processes in Detection and Recognition,* Sensory Intelligence Laboratory, University of Michigan, 1965, will exemplify the principle, though it does not employ speech signals.

The Tanner study was designed to display the ability of an observer to learn to process a complex signal with which he could intuitively be asserted to have had little or no experience. The signal to each ear was a one-hundred-millisecond 1,000 Hertz tone with a shaped amplitude. In one ear the amplitude began the signal interval at zero and increased to a maximum at the end of the interval; in the other ear, the amplitude began the interval at its maximum value and diminished to end the interval at zero. To each signal was added a ten-millisecond pulse, superimposed on the ramp signal, at one of four delays after signal interval initiation. The observer was to push a button corresponding to the time position of the pulse. Following each trial, he was given feedback as to what was the correct response. He was paid $0.003 for each correct response and fined $0.001 for each incorrect response. Each observer participated in either 800 or 1000 trials per day and the results of each day's session was plotted as a single point.

One observer moved significantly off chance performance on the second day and by the tenth day was performing about maximally; that is, he did little better with an additional twenty days' trials. However, another observer "sat" at chance for six days and did not reach maximum performance until

For other types of measures of linguistic performance, it seems that no meaningful dichotomy can be drawn between competence and performance. If the task is one for which the subject must sample his own internal storage and in which he can be considered to have had hundreds of thousands of practice trials, it must be assumed that he samples, from whatever the experimental instructions lead him to consider his sampling set, in a way he has long ago learned will maximize his harvest of information from the message or provide his best guess as to the appropriate response. He should demonstrate the same performance for a task aimed at assessing either performance or competence.

In other words, the first kind of definitional difference proposed for the two concepts asserts that performance is an estimate of present functioning, which for many tasks can be improved with practice. One can obtain an estimate that will be stable, however, only if he does not alert the subject to the fact that the routine payoff matrix, which has previously determined the performance of the subject, has altered in this experiment. If the subject knows what is being appraised, he will begin to improve in performance thus precluding any stable estimate of his performance. The final estimate, when performance has reached some plateau imposed by the limitations of the subject and/or the experiment, can be considered to define competence. A performance measure will be stable if it can be derived, and a competence measure cannot be derived without first training the subject to maximize his processing of the linguistic material. We have already indicated that this latter imposes on the experimenter the task of providing high payoff for maximizing performance and giving the subject a large number of training trials.

There are other tasks for which any subject can be considered to be in such familiar territory and so motivated that it must be assumed (though one can always perform the experiment to see for himself) that the subject is operating as efficiently as he can for the perceived conditions, so that his performance will already have reached his competence plateau.

On the Uses of Normal and Non-Normal Subjects

The above line of reasoning, it seems to me, provides the strongest argument for not applying results from persons who hear normally in typical speech recognition tasks to results to be expected from persons

---

he had participated in approximately 35,000 trials, each with immediate feedback and with a significant monetary advantage for improving performance.

with some loss in their ability to hear speech. For tests of monosyllabic word recognition, the normal hearing subject (at least one as highly verbally and linguistically trained as our typical normal subject—the college sophomore) must be assumed to be capable of processing for maximal advantage in his use of acoustic cues like those he routinely processes. Study after study serves as witness to his ability to resist signal deteriorations of virtually all varieties. This is not necessarily true, however, for the person with a hearing loss for speech, particularly one that has occurred subsequent to his learning of speech and language (to his learning to recognize and process speech cues) in the sense that with normal hearing he not only mastered the rules and the substantive content but also that he had thousands upon thousands of trials in the use of both. This hearing-handicapped person now has the confusion of a set of rules for using acoustic cues to derive the bases of his interpretations of signals into meaningful messages, but a partially or completely altered set of cues. He learned his rules at a time when he was processing speech inputs through a normal system, but his rules are for the cues he heard with the normal system. Now he gets different or altered cues that do not work well under the system of old rules and may not be adequate for any reasonable speech recognition using any set of rules he can change to.

The reader is probably aware that these last few sentences have a loaded assumption underlying them, which is that speech exists only probabilistically in the acoustic waveform. This means that it cannot be specified absolutely and uniquely, and one's ability to understand a spoken message is partially determined by his expectations about that message. The argument is implicit in the proposed model of speech communication and serves as a source for generating additional studies significant to our understanding of speech as a sound signal.

One of the components of speech communication is a question of the criteria for appropriate (acceptable) variance in the sounds of speech, be they phonemes, syllables, or whatever. Vowels are less constrained in physiological placement than consonants so that phonological theory should predict their susceptibility to early production at some acceptable level of precision, with the later production of consonants being ordered by the difficulty in achieving the requisite articulatory precision. By this latter term is meant the necessary limitation on the variance of the productions as well as the appropriate mean placement. Perhaps we could even discover the orderliness of that processing by evaluating the achievement of some criterion-production competence for linguistically distinctive features or something like them.

What we might consider the necessary production variance is related to the criteria imposed (for example, aspiration in prevocalic unclustered voiceless plosive but not in postvocalic nor in prevocalic clustered). The model asserts that the appropriate way to view adequacy of production is not as a production distribution at all, but rather as a reception distribution. It is the unified perception that unites varying productions because the decision process wipes out the differences in aspiration that sort them phonetically. One must deal with the problem within the realization that the perceptual cues are culturally bound so that some cultures make a cue significant only phonetically, another culture (perhaps speaking the same "language") makes it a more important cue of phonemic significance. Therefore, if one wishes to view production variance, he must first free himself of his linguistic assumptions, his expectations, and his phonemic perceptions, and only then, when he is building observations rather than reaching decisions on observations with respect to fences, can he learn something about constraints on production variance.

Two New Performance Measures

The most common measure used in speech and hearing is percentage correct (which we shall refer to as P(C)). The measure is applicable to procedures using various magnitudes of materials, is easily interpreted, and is widely understood (at least in part). Unfortunately, it is also very wasteful and too often, much less useful than we take it to be.

The P(C) is wasteful because it dismisses all correct data as being equally correct and all incorrect data as being equally incorrect. There is no way to give a higher score to an answer about which we are positive than one which is only a lucky guess. And there is no information in any incorrect response so that if, for example, we are doing an experiment where a subject is performing at 40 percent correct, we are throwing away 60 percent of our data (and wasting 60 percent of the experimental time).

If we compare individual scores by considering only their rank orders, then we are using the P(C) score correctly. If we have reason to consider that the test items are homogeneous, then we can also meaningfully cite the size of a P(C) difference and consider, for example, that a subject with a score of 70 percent is as much superior to another with a score of 63 percent as the latter is superior to yet a third subject with a score of 56 percent. We frequently draw these kinds of conclusions but much less frequently could we justify them if challenged to do so. Where test items are not interchangeable, P(C) should not be applied in this latter manner.

We invite the reader to evaluate two alternatives that might prove useful adjunctive or substitute measures for P(C). Both use all the data rather than only those the subject gets correctly, but they use them in different ways. Unfortunately, neither directly weights a measure by the subject's confidence in it although both reflect aspects of the underlying discriminability. The first of these measures is Percentage Transmitted Information $P(\hat{T})$ and the other is an index we shall call A-prime (A').

PERCENTAGE TRANSMITTED INFORMATION

This first alternative measure has a potential for being highly useful as a device for measuring progress in therapy, as well as for a variety of other tasks. The measure should be particularly good for evaluating therapeutic progress because first, it is sensitive to the consistency (or lack of consistency) of response behaviors and second, it makes very few demands on assumptions that should be met for legitimate application of the measure. The implication of requiring virtually no parameters for application is that the user can combine and categorize his data in any way he pleases, or in every way he pleases, and do additional analyses. But more of this later.

Percentage transmitted information $P(\hat{T})$ is derived from two other terms ($\hat{T}$ and H(x)) so we will deal with these two unknown quantities and some general aspects of measuring information.[28] Information, also called Uncertainty, is defined as a property of a set of potential messages or potential signals, and it increases as the number of possible messages increases. If I am awaiting a message which I know will be either *A* or *B*, then I don't have very much uncertainty about what the message is if poorly transmitted—it's either *A* or *B*. But if the message can be any of a thousand messages, then a poor transmission leaves me with greater uncertainty, as I don't know which of the thousand messages it was.

Information transmission deals with a calculation of the uncertainty or information about a message prior to its delivery (H(x), called H of x), and the uncertainty, if any, after its delivery ($H_y(x)$, called H of x, given y). The difference between the two uncertainties is the information transmitted ($\hat{T}$), where $\hat{T} = H(x) - H_y(x)$. The measure, $100\{1 - [\hat{T}/H(x)]\}\%$, is an estimate of the percentage information.

The measure assumes that prior uncertainties can be calculated, that each message is delivered many times and that the responder's performance is better than all wrong but less good than all correct. Calculation procedures for use of uncertainty analysis are available in many

[28] Garner, *Uncertainty and Structure as Psychological Concepts.*

locations (for example, in Garner [29]). The utility of the procedure is potentially high because the measure is particularly sensitive to ambiguity and equivocation in the listener. Ambiguity is expressed as his use of many different response labels for repeated deliveries of the same signal. Equivocation is expressed as the use of the same response label for different signals. Both are reflected in a signal x response matrix as a scattering of responses into incorrect cell locations.

As an item of interest, the metric is not sensitive to whether signals are correctly identified, only that they be consistently and differentially identified, and for purposes of therapeutic evaluation the matter is of small importance. If a patient learns consistent discrimination and identification, the label he uses can be altered easily to the correct one.

RESPONSE DISCRIMINATION

The second new metric is not nearly as sensitive to changes in the numbers going into it, but it does have the advantage of being influenced by the scatter of the data and by whether the responses were correct. In this sense, it contains the advantages of both $P(C)$ and $P(\hat{T})$. The example to be used concerns training of hearing-handicapped children, but this same metric has been applied to the speech of esophageal (alaryngeal) adults and, in the view of the author, the quantification procedure is more important for the reader to grasp than the particular application used in the example.

The concern in the specific research project was to find a means of quantifying the performance of individual hearing-handicapped children discriminating phonemically or linquistically distinctive features. The goal was to discover a procedure that could be used to focus on sharpening the auditory discrimination of these children, all auditorially oriented, so that they could be drilled on those sounds requiring such practice so long, but only so long, as additional practice would benefit the child.[30]

The standard measure of percentage correct identification was rejected as a measure of performance, because it was obvious with these youngsters, as with other patients of any age, that a particular person

[29] Garner, *Uncertainty and Structure as Psychological Concepts.*

[30] M. C. Schultz and A. W. Kraat, "Lack of Perceptual Reality of the Phoneme for Hearing-Handicapped Children," *Language and Speech*, 12 (1971), 178-186, and, by the same authors, "A Metric for Evaluating Therapy with the Hearing-Impaired," *Journal of Speech and Hearing Disorders*, 35 (1970), 37–43.

may, with increasing amounts of practice, show no improvement in percentage correct recognitions of, for example, a given phoneme, but might continue to show a reduction in those sounds he was mistaking for the sound under test. That is, his hit rate may not be improving but his false alarm rate may be diminishing (he reduces his equivocation), and this result would be significant for us though it would not be reflected in a percentage correct measure of the sound under test (of course, it would be found in an increasing P(C) score for the sound previously being mis-identified). What we required was some performance index reflecting both hits and false alarms, and offering a means of comparing different results.

The metric of the theory of signal detectability employs just such a measure. For simple signals and simple tasks (for example, a two-alternative forced-choice task for tonal signals of given sound pressure level and duration in a white-noise background) one can construct a function of all points of equivalent performance (equivalent sensitivity) with the variable being the strategy of the listener—his willingness to

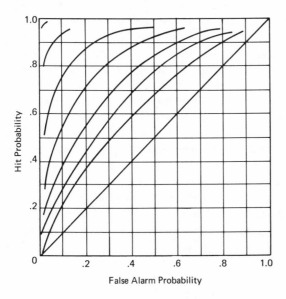

FIGURE 27. *Operating characteristics for distributions with varying degrees of distinctiveness.*

guess about the presence of the signal in a given interval. This function, plotted in a two-dimensional space of proportion of hits by proportion of false alarms, is displayed as Figure 27. The shape of the function, called an operating characteristic, is a reflection of the psychological processes underlying the decision processing so that the user must have a theoretical basis for predicting the shape of the operating characteristic or he must derive the function empirically.

Because of the complexity of speech, we were not prepared to impute any particular set of psychological processing activities nor, for this experiment, were we prepared to derive the curve empirically. (An experimenter could, of course, do so by performing the task repeatedly with the same subjects, each time altering the strategy of the subject systematically by changing the utilities of particular decisions to the subject.) Therefore we had to settle for an analysis of the behavior that allowed comparisons among repeated measures, expressing both different hit rates and different false alarm rates, but that was free of the assertion of any particular operating characteristic and its associated processing implications. It was obvious that any such index was going to suffer inherent inadequacies; for example, one could use it only to rank order his performance estimates without being able to discuss magnitudes of differences separating the numbers, but even this limited insight would be superior to the measure of percentage correct now typically employed.

The experimental procedure used in the study involved having the children respond to a large number of productions of sets of consonant-vowel (CV) syllables, using a set of eight consonants and two vowels. The child responded by pressing a large button on an eight-button board, and he was given money for his performance. Because of the use of a known set of responses and a forced-choice response procedure, a closed signal-by-response matrix was derived, both for consonants and linguistically distinctive features, separately for each vowel. From these matrices, hit rates and false alarm rates were calculated.

The results, while important, are not our concern; the interested reader can find them elsewhere in print.[31] What is important here is that this approach provided a metric that allowed direct comparisons of performance, sometimes in the face of a changing hit rate, and sometimes in the face of a changing false-alarm rate. This gave a simple index of the patient's performance that could be used to plot his discrimination upon entering therapy and at various stages during therapy. As long as he continued to show improvement he could remain with the training procedure, the procedures being altered when his performance ceased showing improvement. (This argument is not inconsistent with the previous discussion of performance versus competence. What is being claimed here is that a patient may achieve a plateau with a procedure at some

---

[31] Schultz and Kraat, "Lack of Perceptual Reality," and "A Metric for Evaluating Therapy."

lower terminal behavior than he would with a more potent therapy; additionally, one can obtain estimates of his locus on the learning curve as he progresses in therapy, even though we are aware that the estimates will not be as stable—show as little variance—as will terminal estimates of behavioral achievement.) Needless to say, the use of a total set of speech sounds would have allowed a determination of the loci of therapeutic need, with respect to the sounds that were most interfering with his perception.[32]

Two expanding arcs of research arise from this example, On the one hand, the metric itself can be applied in a variety of studies requiring some measure of production or reception performance with greater utility than percentage correct allows. We have discussed in several ways why percentage correct confounds both sensitivity and decision strategy and is, therefore, grossly inadequate as an index of almost any performance of interest by the clinical subject. This clinical patient, whether his problem is speech or hearing, is sharply aware of his own difficulties, so we cannot presume to understand his perceptions a priori. Therefore, we cannot presume to be able to separate his decision strategies from his sensitivity without either systematic exploration of each or the use of a measure for either that is not contaminated by the influence of the other.

The other area of research is to undertake systematic studies designed to derive operating characteristics for various types of speech signals. Several steps would follow the generation of these functions. First would be to attempt evaluation of the psychological processes by exploration of both the constants and the variables of the equations of the functions empirically derived. In addition, one could explore the relationships existing among the operating characteristics for various classes of speech signals, the influence of various speech or hearing problems on such operating characteristics as we do find, and so forth.

[32] The metric was derived by I. Pollack and D. A. Norman, "A Non-Parametric Analysis of Recognition Experiments," *Phychonomic Sciences*, 1 (1964), 125–126. The tables that are used to derive the Pollack-Norman index (called A') from the obtained hit and false alarm rates are published in a laboratory report from the Speech and Hearing Sciences Laboratory of the Indiana University Speech and Hearing Center.

Epilogue

The profession of speech pathology and audiology is going through a revolution. So far it has been a quiet revolution but it may soon become very noisy—at least vocally. It is a revolution in methods and techniques, and it comes about, as is true of most revolutions, because of both internal and external pressures.

The external pressures arise because our society is highly communicative, so that good communication ability is considered necessary and people want it enough to be willing to pay for it. This creates a great demand for our services as professionals, which we consider good because our salaries increase and with them our status in the community. And this gives rise to the internal pressures.

The internal pressures have to do with training. If we need more professionals, then training programs must expand—as, indeed, they have been doing—to turn out more clinicians to meet the increased demand for services. However, at the same time that the demand for therapy increases, the profession has moved toward reducing the proportion of its graduating student population entering therapy. While we have been increasing our student population, we have been bleeding a large segment into audiological diagnosis, an increasing number into research, and we have branched into new areas of exploration (for example, the culturally disadvantaged, aphasia). In addition, at a time when more and more therapists are required, we are making our training programs longer and raising our standards—making it more difficult to get into training and then more difficult to finish training.

And so we have a revolution in the making—a series of external pressures toward increasing training productivity and a series of counterproductive offshoots from training (counterproductive only in the sense that they are not positive responses aimed at relieving the external pressures).

The revolution in the making is in the form of technologies increasing economies of training and technologies for increasing therapy efficiency. Some of these techniques are with us now (for example, video-tape recording/reproduction for clinical teaching) whereas others are only barely on the horizon (for example, computerized diagnostics), but they, or some equally economical alternatives, will come because the pressures are inexorable and growing.

If these insights are accurate, then we must master our own house, determine where technologies increasing our efficiency are appropriately to be introduced and where not, and move willingly into discovering and introducing new technologies as rapidly as possible.

This work has been addressed to the attempt to formalize aspects of certain clinical processes so that they might be seen stripped of many of the complexities that typically make for so much difficulty in analyzing them. Some ideas about applications of new technologies have also been introduced.

It may be that the reader will find fault both with the model and the portions of clinical activities into which I assert we can introduce new technologies. The argument is healthy and welcome because it will aid us in seeing our problems and our options for solutions, hopefully more clearly than we see them now.

But the revolution is already upon us and we only hope to channel and focus it—we cannot prevent it.

Bibliography

General

ATTNEAVE, F., *Applications of Information Theory to Psychology*. New York, Holt, 1959

BATTEAU, D. W., R. L. PLANTE, R. H. SPENCER, W. E. LYLE, *Auditory Perception*. China Lake, Calif., U.S. Naval Ordinance Test Station, Contract No. N123–(60530) 35401A, United Research Inc., Cambridge, October 1964.

BRUNER, J., *Toward a Theory of Instruction*. Cambridge, Harvard University Press (Belknap Press), 1966.

BUGELSKI, B. R., *The Psychology of Learning Applied to Teaching*. Indianapolis, Bobbs-Merrill, 1964.

CHOMSKY, N., Review of B. F. Skinner's, *Verbal Behavior, Language*, 35 (1959), 26–58.

———, *Aspects of the Theory of Syntax*. Cambridge, MIT Press, 1965.

GARNER, W. R., *Uncertainty & Structure as Psychological Concepts*. New York, Wiley, 1962.

GOFFMAN, ERVING, *The Presentation of Self in Everyday Life*. Garden City, Doubleday, Anchor Books, 1959.

GOLDIAMOND, I., "Perception," in *The Experimental Foundations of Clinical Psychology*, ed. A. Bachrach. New York, Basic Books, 1963.

——— and W. F. HAWKINS, "Vexierversuch: The Log Relationship Between Word-Frequency and Recognition Obtained in the Absence of Stimulus Words," *Journal of Experimental Psychology*, 56 (1958), 456–463.

GUTTMAN, N., "Measurement of Articulatory Merit," *Journal of Speech and Hearing Research*, 9 (1966), 323–339.

———, "A Nomogram for the Articulatory Product," *Journal of Speech and Hearing Research*, 10 (1967), 311–312.

HALL, E. T., *The Silent Language*. Greenwich, Conn., Fawcett, 1966.

167

HEYNS, R. W. and R. LIPPITT, "Systematic Observational Techniques," in *Handbook of Social Psychology*, ed. G. Lindzey. Cambridge, Addison and Wesley, 1954.

HOLLAND, J. G., and B. F. SKINNER, *Analysis of Behavior: Programmed Instruction*. New York, McGraw-Hill, 1961.

HOMME, L. E., "Contiguity Theory & Contingency Management," *The Psychological Record*, 16 (1966), 233–241.

MANNHEIM, K., *Ideology & Utopia*. New York, Harcourt, 1966.

NORMAN, D. A., *Memory and Attention: An introduction to human information processing*. New York, Wiley, 1969.

PREMACK, D., "Reinforcement Theory," in *Nebraska Symposium on Motivation*, ed. D. Levine. Lincoln, University of Nebraska Press, 1965.

ROGERS, C., *On Becoming a Person*. Boston, Houghton Mifflin, 1961.

WATANABE, S., "Information-Theoretical Aspects of Inductive and Deductive Inferences," *IBM Journal of Research & Development*, 14 (1960), 208–231.

Statistical Decision Theory and the Theory of Signal Detectability

ATTNEAVE, F., *Applications of Information Theory to Psychology*. New York, Holt, 1959.

BROSS, I. J. D., *Design For Decision*. New York, Free Press, 1953.

EDWARDS, W. and A. TVERSKY, eds., *Decision Making*. Baltimore, Penguin Books, Inc., 1967.

EGAN, J. P., *Signal Detection Theory and Psychophysics: A Topical Bibliography*. Technical Report, Grant AF–AFOSR–548–67, Hearing and Communication Laboratory, Indiana University, June 1967.

GARNER, W. R., *Uncertainty & Structure as Psychological Concepts*. New York, Wiley, 1962.

GREEN, D. M. and J. A. SWETS, *Signal Detection Theory and Psychophysics*. New York, Wiley, 1966.

POLLACK, I. and D. NORMAN, "A Non-Parametric Analysis of Recognition Experiments," *Psychonomic Sciences*, 1 (1964), 125–126.

SHANNON, C. E., "The Mathematical Theory of Communication," in C. E. Shannon and W. Weaver, *The Mathematical Theory of Communication*. Urbana, University of Illinois Press, 1964.

SWETS, J. A., "Is There A Sensory Threshold?" *Science*, 134 (1961), 168–177.

———, ed., *Signal Detection and Recognition in Human Observers*. New York, Wiley, 1964.

TANNER, W. P., JR., "On the Design of Psychophysical Experiments," in *Information Theory in Psychology,* ed. H. Quastler. Glencoe, Free Press, 1955.

——, "Physiological Implications of Psychophysical Data," in *Signal Detection and Recognition in Human Observers,* ed. J. A. Swets, New York, Wiley, 1964.

——, *Statistical Decision Processes in Detection & Recognition.* University of Michigan, Sensory Intelligence Laboratory, 1965.

Models

BERMAN, M., W. P. TANNER, JR., and M. C. SCHULTZ, "Intelligibility and Intelligence of Speech," *Journal of the Acoustical Society of America,* in press.

BRODBECK, M., "Models, Meaning & Theories," in *Symposium on Sociological Theory,* ed. L. Gross. Evanston, Row, Peterson, 1959.

BROSS, I. J. D., *Design for Decision.* New York, Free Press, 1953.

FAIRBANKS, G., *Experimental Phonetics: Selected Articles.* Urbana, University of Illinois Press, 1966.

GARNER, W. R., *Uncertainty & Structure as Psychological Concepts.* New York, Wiley, 1962.

GIULIANO, V. E., "Analog networks for word association," *IEEE Transactions on Military Electronics* (1963), MIL–7, 221–225.

HOMME, L. E., "Contiguity Theory & Contingency Management," *The Psychological Record,* 16 (1966), 233–241.

MYSAK, E., *Speech Pathology & Feedback Theory.* Springfield, Thomas, 1966.

NORMAN, D. A., *Memory and Attention: An introduction to human information processing.* New York, Wiley, 1969.

RIGG, K. E. and J. C., *Behavioral Engineering: Adaptation of Emotional Behavior.* Report 69–001, Communications Research Laboratory, Department of Speech, New Mexico State University, January, 1969.

SCHULTZ, M. C., "The Bases of Speech Pathology & Audiology: What are Appropriate Models?" *Journal of Speech and Hearing Disorders,* 37 (1972), in press.

SIDMAN, M., "Operant Techniques," in *Experimental Foundations of Clinical Psychology,* ed. A. J. Bachrach. New York, Basic Books, 1962.

SWETS, J. A., ed., *Signal Detection & Recognition in Human Observers.* New York, Wiley, 1964.

Speech Discrimination, Intelligibility, Recognition

BERMAN, M., W. P. TANNER, JR., and M. C. SCHULTZ, "Intelligibility and Intelligence of Speech," *Journal of Acoustical Society of America,* in press.

EGAN, J. P., "Articulation Testing Methods," *The Laryngoscope,* 58 (1948), 955–991.

FAIRBANKS, G., *Experimental Phonetics: Selected Articles.* Urbana, University of Illinois Press, 1966.

GOLDIAMOND, I. and W. F. HAWKINS, "Vexierversuch: The Log Relationship Between Word-Frequency and Recognition Obtained in the Absence of Stimulus Words," *Journal of Experimental Psychology,* 56 (1958), 456–463.

HEFFLER, A. J. and M. C. SCHULTZ, "Some Implications of Binaural Signal Selection for Hearing Aid Evaluation," *Journal of Speech and Hearing Research,* 7 (1964), 279–289.

SCHULTZ, M. C. and M. BERMAN, "Speech Recognition Behavior in Normals and Otopathological Persons," *Journal of Speech and Hearing Research,* in press.

—— and A. W. KRAAT, "Lack of Perceptual Reality of the Phoneme for Hearing-Handicapped Children," *Language and Speech,* 12 (1972), 178–186.

—— and E. D. SCHUBERT, "A Multiple Choice Discrimination Test (MCDT)," *The Laryngoscope,* 79 (1969), 382–399.

—— and C. S. STREEPY, "The Speech Discrimination Function in Loudness Recruiting Ears," *The Laryngoscope,* 77 (1967), 2114–2127.

SHANNON, C. E., "The Mathematical Theory of Communication," in C. E. Shannon and W. Weaver, *The Mathematical Theory of Communication.* Urbana, University of Illinois Press, 1964.

SPEAKS, C. E., "Synthetic-Sentence Identification and the Receiver Operating Characteristic," *Journal of Speech and Hearing Research,* 10 (1967), 110–119.

SWETS, J. A., ed., *Signal Detection & Recognition in Human Observers.* New York, Wiley, 1964.

Supervision and Clinical Training in Speech and Hearing

ANDERSON, J. and D. KIRTLEY, eds., *Institute on Supervision of Speech and Hearing Programs in the Public Schools.* Bloomington, Indiana University, 1966.

BACKUS, O. and J. BEASLEY, *Speech Therapy with Children.* Boston, Houghton Mifflin, 1951.

BARKER, R. G., et. al., *Adjustment to Physical Handicap and Illness: A Survey of the Social Psychology of Physical Disability.* New York, Social Science Research Council, 1960.

CAPELLA, G., "When a Deaf Person Must Wear a Hearing Aid," *Medical Clinics,* 25 (1955), 95–98.

CONNOR, L. L., "Diagnostic Teaching—The Teacher's New Role," *Volta Review,* 61 (1959), 311–315.

COOPER, E. B., "Client-Clinician Relationships and Concomitant Factors in Stuttering Therapy," *Journal of Speech and Hearing Research,* 9 (1966), 194–207.

DIEDRICH, W., "Use of Video Tape in Teaching Clinical Skills," *Volta Review,* 68 (1966), 644–647.

——, "Analysis of the Clinical Process," *Journal of the Kansas Speech and Hearing Association,* 1969, 1–8.

ERIKSON, E. and C. VAN RIPER, "Demonstration Therapy in University Training Center," *ASHA,* 9 (1967), 33–35.

HAHN, E., "Communication in the Therapy Session: A Point of View," *Journal of Speech and Hearing Disorders,* 25 (1960), 18–23.

——, "Indications for Direct, Non-Direct and Indirect Methods in Speech Correction," *Journal of Speech and Hearing Disorders,* 26 (1961), 230–236.

HALFOND, M. M., "Clinical Supervision: Step-Child in Training," *ASHA,* 6 (1964), 441–444.

MARTIN, E. W., "Client Centered Therapy as a Theoretical Orientation for Speech Therapy," *ASHA,* 5 (1963), 576–578.

NAYLOR, R. V., "Certification and Clinical Practicum" (letter to the Editor) *ASHA,* 4 (1964), 146.

NUTTALL, E. C., "When Should Clinical Practice Begin?" *ASHA,* 2 (1960), 207–208.

PERKINS, W., "Our Profession, What is it? *ASHA,* 4 (1962), 339–344.

—— and R. F. CURLEE, "Causality in Speech Pathology," *Journal of Speech and Hearing Disorders,* 34 (1969), 231–238.

PTACEK, P., "Supportive Personnel as an Extension of the Professional Worker's Nervous System," *ASHA,* 9 (1967), 403–405.

REES, M. and G. L. SMITH, "Supervised School Experience for Student Clinicians," *ASHA,* 9 (1957), 251–256.

SCHULTZ, M. C., "The Bases of Speech Pathology and Audiology: What are Appropriate Models?" *Journal of Speech and Hearing Disorders,* 37 (1972), in press.

SHERMAN, D., "Clinical and Experimental Use of the Iowa Scale of Severity of Stuttering," *Journal of Speech and Hearing Disorders,* 17 (1952), 316–320.

—— and C. E. MOODIE, "Four Psychological Scaling Methods Applied to Articulation Defectiveness," *Journal of Speech and Hearing Disorders,* 20, (1955), 352–358.

SLOANE, H. and B. MACAULAY, *Operant Procedures in Remedial Speech & Language Training.* Boston, Houghton Mifflin, 1968.

STACE, A. C. and A. B. DREXLER, "Special Training for Supervisors of Student Clinicians: What Private Speech and Hearing Centers Do and Think About Training Their Supervisors," *ASHA,* 11 (1969), 318–320.

VAN RIPER, C., "Supervision of Clinical Practice," *ASHA,* 7 (1965), 75–77.

——, "Success and Failure in Speech Therapy," *Journal of Speech and Hearing Disorders,* 31 (1966), 276–279.

WARD, L. M. and E. J. WEBSTER, ('The Training of Clinical Personnel: I. Issues in Conceptualization," *ASHA,* 7 (1965), 38–40.

——, "The Training of Clinical Personnel: II. A Concept of Clinical Preparation," *ASHA,* 7 (1965), 103–106.

Clinical Training of Other Professions

BACHRACH, A. J., ed., *Experimental Foundations of Clinical Psychology.* New York, Basic Books, 1962.

CARKUFF, R. and B. BERENSON, *Beyond Counseling and Therapy.* New York, Holt, 1967.

CONNOR, L. L., "Diagnostic Teaching—The Teacher's New Role," *Volta Review,* 61 (1959), 311–315.

GARDNER, G. G., "The Psychological Relationship," *The Psychological Bulletin,* 61 (1964), 426–439.

HEFFERLINE, R. F., "Learning Theory and Clinical Psychology—An Eventual Symbiosis?" in A. J. Bachrach, *Experimental Foundations.*

HUNT, W. L., "Psychotherapy as a Group Process, "*Journal of General Psychology,* 66 (1962), 61–69.

HUNT, W. A. and N. F. JONES, "Experimental Investigation of Clinical Judgment," in A. J. Bachrach, *Experimental Foundations.*

KENNEDY, A., "Chance and Design in Psychotherapy," *Journal of Mental Sciences,* 106 (1960), 1–16.

MATARAZZO, J. D., "Some Psychotherapists Make Patients Worse!" *International Journal of Psychiatry,* 3 (1967), 156–157.

MEEHL, P. E., *Clinical Versus Statistical Prediction: A Theoretical Analysis and*

A Review of the Literature. Minneapolis, University of Minnesota Press, 1954.

PERCY, W., "The Symbolic Structure of Interpersonal Process," *Psychiatry*, 24 (1961), 39–52.

ROGERS, C. R., "The Therapeutic Relationship: Recent Theory and Research, *Australian Journal of Psychology*, 17 (1956), 95–108.

SCHALOCK, H. D., CLARK SMITH and FRANCES VOGEL, "An Overview of the TEACHING RESEARCH System For the Description of Teacher Behavior in Context," in Anita Simon and E. Gil Boyer, eds., *Mirrors for Behavior: An Anthology of Classroom Observation Instruments*, Vol 12, 1970.

SHANDS, H. C., *Thinking And Psychotherapy: An Inquiry into the Process of Communication*. Cambridge, Harvard University Press, 1960.

SIGAL, J. J., "Symposium—Conditioning Therapy. Operant Conditioning and Some Aspects of the Psychotherapeutic Process," *Journal of the Canadian Psychiatric Association*, 12 (1967), 3–8.

SIMON, ANITA, and E. GIL BOYER, eds. *Mirrors for Behavior: An Anthology of Classroom Observation Instruments*. Vol. 12, 1970.

STRUPP, H. H., "Toward an Analysis of the Therapist's Contribution to the Treatment Process," *Psychiatry*, 22 (1959), 349–362.

THOMAS, E. J., Selected Sociobehavioral Techniques and Principals: an Approach to Interpersonal Helping," *Social Work*, 13 (1968), 12–26.

THORNE, F. C., "The Clinical Method in Science," in *Readings in The Clinical Method in Psychology*, ed. R. I. Watson, New York, Harper, 1949.

TRUAX, C. B., "The Empirical Emphasis in Psychotherapy: A Symposium. Effective Ingredients in Psychotherapy: An Approach to Unraveling the Patient-Therapist Interaction," *Journal of Consulting Psychology*, 10 (1963), 256–263.

TRUAX, C. B. and R. R. CARKUFF, "Experimental Manipulation of Therapeutic Conditions," *Journal of Consulting Psychology*, 29 (1965), 119–124.

——, *Toward Effective Counseling and Psychotherapy: Training and Practice*. Chicago, Aldine, 1967.

ULLMAN, L. and L. KRASNER, *Case Studies in Behavior Modification*. New York, Holt, 1968.

WATSON, R. I., *Readings in the Clinical Method in Psychology*. New York, Harper, 1949.

Speech Pathology and Therapy

BACKUS, O. and J. BEASLEY, *Speech Therapy With Children*. Boston, Houghton Mifflin, 1951.

GARRETT, E. R., *Speech and Language Therapy Under An Automated Stimulus Control System*. Final Report, Project No. 3191, Contract No. OE–6–10–198, New Mexico State University, January 1968.

GUTTMAN, N., "Measurement of Articulatory Merit," *Journal of Speech and Hearing Research,* 9 (1966), 323–339.

———, "A Nomogram for the Articulatory Product," *Journal of Speech and Hearing Research,* 10 (1967), 311–312.

MILISEN, R., "Articulatory Problems," in *Speech Pathology,* ed. R. W. Rieber and R. S. Brubaker. Amsterdam, North-Holland Publishing Co., 1966.

RIGG, K. E. and J. C., *Mod II "S" Meter*. Report 68–002. Communications Research Laboratory, Department of Speech, New Mexico State University, August 1968.

———, *Behavioral Engineering: Adaptation of Emotional Behavior*. Report 69–001, Communications Research Laboratory, Department of Speech, New Mexico State University, January 1969.

SHERMAN, D., "Clinical and Experimental Use of the Iowa Scale of Severity of Stuttering," *Journal of Speech and Hearing Disorders,* 17 (1952), 316–320.

——— and C. E. MOODIE, "Four Psychological Scaling Methods Applied to Articulation Defectiveness," *Journal of Speech and Hearing Disorders,* 20 (1955), 352–358.

SLOANE, H. and B. MACAULAY, *Operant Procedures in Remedial Speech & Language Training*. Boston, Houghton Mifflin, 1968.

Hearing Pathology and Therapy

DAVIS, H., "The Articulation Area and the Social Adequacy Index for Hearing," *The Laryngoscope,* 58 (1948), 761–778.

———, "Information Theory: Three Applications of Information Theory to Research in Hearing," *Journal of Speech and Hearing Disorders,* 17 (1952), 189–197.

——— and S. R. SILVERMAN, *Hearing and Deafness,* third ed. New York, Holt, 1970.

GREENSPAN, C. F. and K. C. POLLACK, "Response Variability and Personality Factors in Automated Audiometry," *Journal of Auditory Research,* 9 (1969), 386–390.

HEFFLER, A. J. and M. C. SCHULTZ, "Some Implications of Binaural Signal Selection for Hearing-Aid Evaluation," *Journal of Speech and Hearing Research,* 7 (1964), 279–289.

RAMSDELL, D. A., "The Psychology of the Hard-of-Hearing and the Deafened Adult," in H. Davis and S. R. Silverman, *Hearing and Deafness.*

RIGG, K. E. and J. C., *Behavioral Engineering: Adaptation of Emotional Behavior.* Report 69–001, Communications Research Laboratory, Department of Speech, New Mexico State University, January 1969.

SCHULTZ, M. C., "Classroom Appraisal of Hearing-Aid Effectiveness, *The Speech Teacher,* 15 (1966), 132–135.

—— and M. BERMAN, "Speech Recognition Behavior in Normals and Otopathological Persons," *Journal of Speech and Hearing Research,* in press.

—— and A. W. KRAAT, "A Metric for Evaluating Therapy with the Hearing Impaired," *Journal of Speech and Hearing Disorders,* 35 (1970), 37–43.

—— and A. W. KRAAT, "Lack of Perceptual Reality of the Phoneme for Hearing-Handicapped Children," *Language and Speech,* 12 (1971), 178–186.

—— and E. D. SCHUBERT, "A Mutiple Choice Discrimination Test (MCDT)," *The Laryngoscope,* 79 (1969), 382–399.

—— and C. S. STREEPY, "The Speech Discrimination Function in Loudness Recruiting Ears," *The Laryngoscope,* 77 (1967), 2114–2127.

SHEPHERT, D. C. and R. GOLDSTEIN, "Relation of Békésy Tracings to Personality and Electrophysiologic Measures," *Journal of Speech and Hearing Research,* 9 (1966), 385–411.

——, "Intrasubject Variability in Amplitude of Békésy Tracings and Its Relation to Measures of Personality," *Journal of Speech and Hearing Research,* 11 (1968), 525–535.

ZERLIN, S., "A new approach to hearing-aid selection," *Journal of Speech and Hearing Research,* 5 (1962), 370–376.

Index